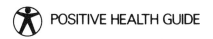 POSITIVE HEALTH GUIDE

THE DIABETICS' DIET BOOK

A new high-fibre eating programme

Dr Jim Mann
and the Oxford Dietetic Group

Roberta Longstaff, SRD
Elizabeth Todd, BSc, SRD
Susan Lousley, BSc (Hons), SRD
Honor Runciman, SRD
Dr Derek Hockaday

Foreword by Dr Arnold Bloom,
Chairman, Executive Council, British Diabetic Association

MARTIN DUNITZ

To all our patients who have taken part in the experiments that have led to the development of our new diet.

© Jim Mann, 1982

First published in the United Kingdom
in 1982 by Martin Dunitz Limited,
London

British Library Cataloguing-in-Publication Data

Mann, Jim
    The diabetics' diet book.–(Positive health guide)
    1. Diabetes–Diet therapy–Recipes
    I. Title II. Oxford Dietetic Group III. Series
    641.5'6314   RC662
    ISBN 0-906348-34-X
    ISBN 0-906348-35-8 Pbk

Designed by Anita Ruddell
Cover photograph by Roger Phillips
Inside photographs by Rob Matheson
Food prepared by Hilary Walden
Props provided by The Reject Shop, King's Road, London;
    and Sally Dawson

Phototypeset in Garamond by Bookens, Saffron Walden, Essex
Printed in Singapore by Tien Wah Press (Pte) Ltd.

Cover photograph shows Italian vegetable soup, Salade Niçoise, Vegetarian bean paella, Quick wholemeal bread and Sparkling fruit salad.

Dr Jim Mann is University Lecturer in Social and Community Medicine at Oxford University and is Honorary Consultant Physician at the Radcliffe Infirmary and John Radcliffe Hospital in Oxford. He began his research into diabetic diets, aided by numerous colleagues, in 1972. Much of his research has involved the comparison of new high-fibre diets with the old-fashioned low-carbohydrate, high-fat diabetic diets. He and his team have confirmed the success of their new diet in controlling blood sugar by monitoring its effects over several years in large numbers of patients.

The Oxford Dietetic Group comprises: **Dr Jim Mann**; **Roberta Longstaff**, Area Dietitian, Oxfordshire Area Health Authority; **Elizabeth Todd**, Chief Dietitian, John Radcliffe Hospital, Oxford; **Susan Lousley**, Chief Dietitian, Radcliffe Infirmary, Oxford; **Honor Runciman**, Community Dietitian, Oxfordshire Area Health Authority; and **Dr Derek Hockaday**, Consultant Physician at the Radcliffe Infirmary and the John Radcliffe Hospital, Oxford.

Authors' acknowledgements
We are grateful to our diabetic patients for their participation in our research, to the British Diabetic Association for financial support, and to Mrs Anne Reeve and Mrs Jill Gemmell for typing the manuscript. Many of our colleagues have provided ideas and encouragement but the following have played key roles in the research: Richard Simpson, Hugh Simpson and David Jones (Research Fellows); Jane Eaton and Moira Geekie (Dietitians); Robin Carter, Richard Jelfs and Karen Barker (Laboratory Scientific Officers); and Elaine Cassels and Pam Slaughter (Nursing Sisters).

Food analysis figures are based on *McCance and Widdowson's The Composition of Foods* (4th rev ed) by A.A. Paul and D.A.T. Southgate; and *Food Composition Tables for Use in East Asia* by the Food and Agriculture Organization.

FOREWORD

Arnold Bloom, MD, FRCP
Chairman, Executive Council, British Diabetic Association

All the experts agree that diet plays an important role in the treatment of diabetes, but the nature of the diet has until recently undergone very little critical inspection. Before the advent of insulin in 1922, the only diet which would prolong life for those with acute diabetes was one of virtual starvation; the less food the better. This attitude undoubtedly coloured the approach to diets thereafter, which were complicated, pernickety and almost impossible for most diabetics to follow with ease – as every investigation into patients' eating patterns showed. These diets were relatively high in fat and protein and low in both starchy and sugary carbohydrate.

It was high time for an intelligent reassessment of the diabetic diet, based not solely on chemical analyses made in the laboratory but on studies on those with diabetes. Such studies have now been undertaken, notably at Oxford, and Dr Mann and the Oxford Dietetic Group are to be complimented on the development of their high-fibre, low-fat diet and on the production of this book, based on sound principles, common-sense and a thorough knowledge of people with diabetes. It is a significant step forward.

CONTENTS

INTRODUCTION

This book has been written at the request of many of our patients and colleagues, both doctors and dietitians. In many diabetic clinics throughout the developed world patients are advised to take a restricted-carbohydrate diet not very different from that which has been in use for several hundred years. Yet in some countries (Japan, for example) diabetics have quite high intakes of starchy carbohydrate; and in such countries diabetes appears to be at least as well controlled as in Britain, North America and Australia, and certainly coronary heart disease occurs less frequently.

Ever since the 1920s a small number of doctors in Britain and North America have suggested that a high starchy carbohydrate diet may be beneficial for the majority of diabetics. In Oxford in England we and others have pursued some of these ideas and have evolved a diet containing substantially more starchy carbohydrate and fibre than is currently generally recommended to diabetics.

Our research has confirmed that on this high-fibre diet blood sugar levels are lower than on the traditional restricted-carbohydrate diet; and likewise blood fat levels are reduced. Furthermore, there is the hope that this improvement in day-to-day diabetic control might in the long term help to reduce the risk of diabetic complications.

Formal recognition for the new diabetic diet came in 1981 when the British Diabetic Association revised its dietary recommendations; the Association now advises a diet very similar to the one in this book.

In Part I, The Diet, we explain the thinking behind our new approach and then show you – whether you are dependent on insulin or not – exactly how to convert your present diet to this healthier and more wholesome pattern of eating. Part II features 145 tried and tested recipes – from snacks and salads to main courses and desserts – most being high in fibre. Each one is accompanied by the nutritional details which will enable you to put our diet plan, explained in Part I, simply into practice.

If you are at present on a low-carbohydrate diet and if you are eating chiefly white bread and refined cereal foods, the foods we are recommending will represent a substantial change in cooking and eating habits. However, almost without exception we have found that those who have tried our kind of wholesome diet soon decide that this is a far tastier and more appetizing pattern of eating and very few ever want to return to their old ways. You will find that our high-fibre diabetic diet is no more expensive than any other, and one of its most important aspects is that it can easily be adapted for the whole family, not just the diabetic. In fact there is a lot of evidence to suggest that it is a far healthier diet than is followed at present by the majority of people in the developed world.

One important word of caution before we begin: the book is not intended to be a do-it-yourself diabetic diet manual. In it we are advocating what will probably be for you a major change in eating habits, and as with any other such alteration in your lifestyle this should only be undertaken in full consultation with your doctor, dietitian or nurse.

PART I

The Diet

What is diabetes?

Most readers will know a great deal about diabetes, but we must make quite sure we are all talking about the same thing before getting down to details of diet.

All forms of diabetes result from a lack of effective insulin. Insulin is one of the most important hormones of the body and is produced by the pancreas. It is responsible for dealing with sugar once it has been absorbed into the bloodstream from the intestines, and has several other roles in helping to maintain normal body function. Consequently lack of insulin results not only in a build-up of sugar in the bloodstream with spill-over into the urine, but also in several other changes in the body's metabolism.

Maturity-onset diabetes

There are two main types of diabetes. The most common is known as maturity-onset diabetes because it nearly always starts in middle age. You might also have heard it called non-insulin dependent diabetes mellitus (NIDDM, for short). People with this condition are almost invariably a little, and quite often very, overweight. They rarely need insulin and the treatment is either diet alone or diet and pills. In maturity-onset diabetes insulin is produced by the pancreas but is ineffective. The condition may show itself by causing a wide variety of symptoms which tend to come on over a period of weeks or months: thirst, the passing of large quantities of urine, hunger, weight loss, blurred vision, feeling generally off-colour, tingling of the fingers and toes, and repeated infections. A person developing diabetes may have one or more of them. Sometimes the symptoms are mild but the diabetes may still be causing undesirable effects in the body.

Juvenile-onset diabetes

Also known as insulin dependent diabetes mellitus (IDDM), this is a less common condition which occurs because the pancreas completely loses its ability to produce insulin. This happens almost exclusively in young people, but it can occur at any age. The symptoms are similar to those for maturity-onset diabetes but they tend to develop much more quickly and to be more severe, leading occasionally to unconsciousness if diabetes is not diagnosed and treated soon enough. Although diet plays an important part in treatment, insulin by injection is essential for all people with this condition.

Diabetes is one of the commonest medical conditions in Westernized countries and for both types diet is one of the most important aspects of treatment. Although there have been many major advances in the treatment of diabetes since the discovery of insulin in the 1920s, there is still no cure. Once diabetes has been diagnosed, diabetics will need to pay attention to their diet for the rest of their lives. This book aims to take some of the tedium out of this aspect of diabetes and to show how it can be turned into an enjoyable and creative experience.

Diabetic diets: a new direction

Is the customary restricted-carbohydrate diet necessary?
There are two forms of carbohydrate – sugars and starches – and both are useful sources of energy. Sugars, which are mostly consumed in the form of sucrose (table sugar) in tea, coffee, cakes and so on are sweet and provide energy rapidly. These foods provide a useful source of energy when the diabetic needs an emergency supply, but on the whole they should be avoided. Starches, which come mainly from cereals and vegetables, provide a better, longer-lasting source of energy, as they are digested slowly. The amount of energy provided by carbohydrate – or indeed any other type of food – is usually measured in calories (Cals), although in some countries kilojoules (kJ) are preferred. (In the book we shall be talking in terms of calories, although for specific amounts of energy the kilojoule equivalent is given where appropriate.)

From earliest times dietary advice for diabetics has been based on the most noticeable feature of the disease: the sugary urine. Because of this excess of sugar, diabetics have been advised to exclude all sweet foods from their diet and to restrict all other carbohydrate-containing foods, which are broken down to a form of sugar by the digestive system. During the last two centuries diets have been modified but even today most diabetics are on a carbohydrate-restricted diet. We have found that although recommended starchy carbohydrate intake for diabetics is currently about 40 per cent of total daily calories, many have much less, often not much more than 30 per cent (as compared with the average Western total carbohydrate intake as starches and sugars of nearly 50 per cent).

Research has shown, however, that diets high in starchy carbohydrate might actually improve blood sugar levels in diabetics and protect against diabetes and its complications.

Over the last eight years Dr James W. Anderson has been one of the pioneers in the use of such diets in the treatment of diabetes in Lexington, Kentucky. He and his colleagues gave maturity-onset diabetics diets in which starchy carbohydrate provided as much as 70 per cent of the total daily calories. In almost all patients there was an improvement in diabetic control and in many cases they found that they were able to reduce the patient's dose of pills. It is clear from Dr Anderson's and others' research that a low-carbohydrate diet is unnecessary for diabetics. The diets used by his group are high in starch but not in sugar. Most of the carbohydrate is derived from cereal and vegetable sources and therefore also contains quite large quantities of dietary fibre. This brings us to the next consideration: just how important is dietary fibre in diabetes?

Improved diabetic control with dietary fibre

Most cereals, vegetables and fruits contain a substance which is not digested or absorbed by the intestine. This substance forms the cell wall of the plant and provides its rigid structure. It is known as roughage or dietary fibre. Common foods that contain a substantial amount of fibre come from unrefined cereals. These foods are wholemeal bread, wholemeal biscuits, wholegrain breakfast cereals, oat biscuits, brown rice and wholegrain pasta. Others come from various kinds of beans: haricot, red kidney, and lima beans, for example.

It is now generally accepted by the medical profession that a generous intake of dietary fibre is one of the best measures against constipation and many other diseases of the bowel. Dr Hugh Trowell was probably the first person to suggest that fibre might also protect against diabetes. He pointed out that between 1941 and 1954 the number of diabetic deaths in Britain fell to half the previous rate, and that this fall coincided with the compulsory use of high-fibre National Flour which contained appreciably more dietary fibre than white flour. Although sugar and fat consumption in Britain rose during the 1950s to levels greater than before the War, diabetes death rates went on falling until 1954, the year in which high-fibre National Flour became no longer compulsory. He suggested on the basis of this and other evidence that a lack of fibre in the diet may be much more important as a contributory cause in diabetes than an excess of sugar as had previously been believed.

So, does dietary fibre have a role in the treatment of diabetes? We have found that it does; and the reason why is tied up with the question of blood sugar control. When sugars are digested on their own by diabetics it is difficult for them to cope with the resultant sudden increase in blood sugar, so if a diabetic diet contains large amounts of sugar it is impossible to achieve good diabetic control.

As we have seen, starches release their energy more slowly

than sugars; they contain strings of sugar molecules bound together which must be broken down in the bowel before being absorbed. This means that they reach the bloodstream more slowly and the available insulin can cope rather better, resulting in a more satisfactory degree of diabetic control. Fibre in foods slows the absorption of sugar even further and so a diet which is high in fibre and starchy foods provides the best chance of achieving really good control of your diabetes. Leguminous fibre (from various dried beans), which forms a gummy solution when mixed with water, tends to improve diabetic control to a greater extent than fibre from cereals and vegetables.

In Oxford we have developed a diet for diabetics in which starchy carbohydrate provides about 50–60 per cent of total daily calorie intake. The carbohydrate is derived from cereals, vegetables, beans and fruit and so the diet is also high in dietary fibre. We have found that blood sugar levels are better throughout the day for all our patients on this diet – whether they have juvenile- or maturity-onset diabetes – compared with when they were eating the old-fashioned carbohydrate-restricted diet, as long as they do not increase the number of calories consumed each day.

We will be explaining how to follow our diet plan on pages 16 to 34, and in Part II you will find the recipes for the dishes which we recommend to our diabetic patients. Although a few found the meals very filling at first, nearly all quickly adapted

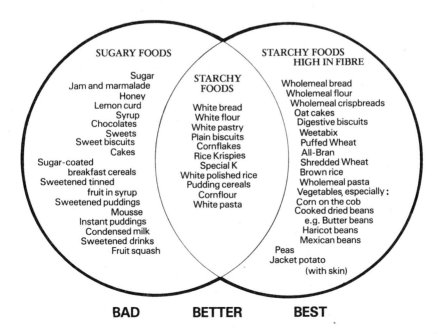

SUGARY FOODS

STARCHY FOODS HIGH IN FIBRE

Sugar
Jam and marmalade
Honey
Lemon curd
Syrup
Chocolates
Sweets
Sweet biscuits
Cakes
Sugar-coated
breakfast cereals
Sweetened tinned
fruit in syrup
Sweetened puddings
Mousse
Instant puddings
Condensed milk
Sweetened drinks
Fruit squash

STARCHY FOODS

White bread
White flour
White pastry
Plain biscuits
Cornflakes
Rice Krispies
Special K
White polished rice
Pudding cereals
Cornflour
White pasta

Wholemeal bread
Wholemeal flour
Wholemeal crispbreads
Oat cakes
Digestive biscuits
Weetabix
Puffed Wheat
All-Bran
Shredded Wheat
Brown rice
Wholemeal pasta
Vegetables, especially:
Corn on the cob
Cooked dried beans
e.g. Butter beans
Haricot beans
Mexican beans
Peas
Jacket potato
(with skin)

BAD   **BETTER**   **BEST**

and everyone found them delicious! Having extra bulk, fibre-rich food will in fact satisfy your hunger better than refined food, and will thus play a vital role in controlling your weight.

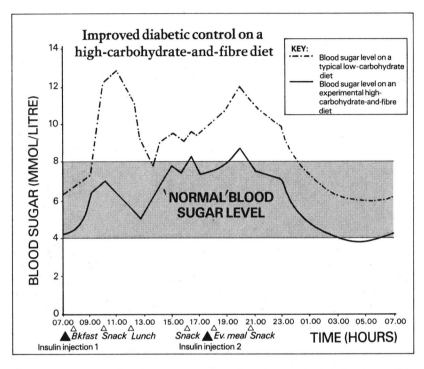

Based on the results of our own research, this graph clearly shows the improvement in blood sugar levels on a high-carbohydrate-and-fibre diet. Values in the shaded area indicate excellent control of diabetes.

Why do diabetics need to control their weight?

There are a number of reasons why people who have developed diabetes should not be overweight. First, with regard to maturity-onset diabetes, we pointed out earlier that insulin was available in the body, but was ineffective. This so-called insulin-resistance is almost certainly associated with obesity and by losing weight the insulin resistance seems at least partly to be overcome. Thus weight reduction is the corner-stone of treatment of maturity-onset diabetes. There are, however, other reasons why diabetics should not be overweight. Raised blood pressure and raised levels of blood fats (cholesterol and triglyceride) are known to be associated with an increased risk of heart disease. Heart disease is a lot more common in diabetics than non-diabetics. It is not known for certain why this should be, but because raised blood pressure and raised levels of blood fats occur frequently in diabetics and, because achieving ideal body weight produces a fall in blood pressure as well as a tendency for blood fats to return to normal levels, people with maturity-onset diabetes should try hard to achieve normal weight.

Although people with juvenile-onset diabetes do not produce insulin it seems that even injected insulin functions less efficiently when people are obese. For this reason and because insulin-requiring diabetics are also at increased risk of coronary heart disease every effort should be made not to be overweight.

Why do you put on weight?
Your body needs energy (calories) from food and drink to perform three types of function. First, to fuel the body processes that are at work when you are resting or even sleeping: for example, breathing, and the pumping of the heart. Then, any form of physical activity, be it eating, typing or walking, requires additional energy. Finally, strenuous exercise like running demands more energy than light exercise.

Your ideal daily energy intake, if you are neither over- nor underweight, should equal the amount of energy expended by your body both at rest and taking exercise. If you achieve this happy state of affairs you are said to be in energy balance, which means that you will neither gain nor lose weight. If on the other hand you consume food and drink which provide more energy than is used in your daily activities, some of the fat, protein and carbohydrate will be converted into body fat and you will start to put on weight.

The only solution if you are gaining weight or are already overweight is to reduce your daily intake of calories. We will be showing you how to go about this on page 18, if you don't need insulin, and on page 24, if you do.

Reduce the amount of fat you eat
Most people think of fat in terms of butter, margarine, oil and lard, and the visible fat on meat. We often forget that there is a less obvious kind of fat: the so-called 'invisible' fats which are found in protein-rich foods such as milk, cheese and meat (even in lean meat – in the muscle where it can't be seen by the naked eye).

Because our new diet contains more than average amounts of cereal and vegetable foods rich in fibre you will find that to maintain ideal body weight it will be necessary to reduce the amount of fat you normally eat. This is not as difficult as it sounds because bulky, high-fibre food is filling and you will not want to eat as much fat, meat and cheese as before. Once you have adjusted the balance of fibre and fat in this way you will probably achieve lower levels of blood cholesterol and this may well decrease your risk of heart disease. In addition, lowering your intake of fat, which has twice the calories of carbohydrate and protein, will help you to reach or maintain your ideal body weight more easily.

Whether or not it is beneficial mostly to use polyunsaturated fat, which will lower cholesterol still further and has other theoretical health advantages, is not completely certain. Our opinion is that it is probably a good idea to have polyunsaturated fat make up about one-third of the total fat in your diet.

Reducing the amount of fat you eat does entail eating less animal protein, which is found in foods such as meat and cheese. Many people think that protein comes only from animal sources but it is important to remember that many vegetables and cereals are high in protein also. Sufficient protein for a day could be provided by eating, for example, either 4 tablespoons of dried beans (soaked and cooked), 4½ large slices of wholemeal bread and just 280 ml/½ pint of skimmed milk; or 1 small fillet of plaice, 4 tablespoons of peas, 2½ slices of wholemeal bread, 1 baked potato with its skin and 1 small 5¼ oz/150 g carton of low-fat yoghurt. There are, of course, many other ways of making up sufficient daily protein intake mainly from vegetable sources. Using the recipes in Part II will go a long way to help you make this change from animal to vegetable protein. When following our diet plan you can be sure that it will provide enough protein for your daily requirements.

How to use this book

Being a diabetic, the chances are that you are used to planning your diet carefully and to calculating the energy and nutritional values of the food you eat, and so following the instructions for the diet plan we are about to describe should present few, if any, problems. If you have not done this sort of thing before, at first glance the diet plan may appear a little daunting. It's rather like reading the rules of a game for the first time: you may not be able to take it all in at once. But don't let that deter you. First read through the sections that apply to your type of diabetes, more than once if necessary, and then go over the details and any questions you have with your medical adviser and dietitian. As when learning a game, you will find that putting the rules into practice is much simpler than you would expect from reading them, especially when you have an expert to guide you.

Here is some useful information about various sections of the book and advice on how to use them.

The recipes (pages 35–118)   These are grouped in chapters according to their contents: soups, salads, baking, and so on. Above each recipe you will find the following nutritional details (per serving): the number of calories/kilojoules (kJ), the number of carbohydrate units, and the amounts of carbohydrate, fibre, fat and protein. The first two items – the calories/kilojoules and carbohydrate units – are particularly important as you will probably need to know these values for all the foods you have on your new diet. The other values are given mainly for doctors and dietitians who will want to refer to these figures in order to verify that you are in fact getting a properly balanced diet. We have included this comprehensive food analysis for another important reason also: if your doctor or dietitian agrees that you should change to high-fibre eating but prefers you to follow their recommended diet plan rather than ours (he or she may want to use a system of exchanges, for instance), then our recipes can still be used. Because we have given the nutritional content of each dish, they can be fitted into any type of high-fibre diabetic diet programme.

We will be recommending that you use as many of these recipes as you can in your diet plan: this means at least one a day, and preferably two.

Appendix 1: Recommended food list   This is a list of foods which together with the recipes should form the basis of your new diet. The foods are neither high in sugar nor fat. Those which are high in fibre are printed in **bold** type for easy reference, and, for diabetics who need insulin, foods which yield 1 unit (10 g) of carbohydrate are marked with an asterisk (see discussion about carbohydrate units on page 25). The foods' calorie and kiljoule values, which all diabetics will need to know, are also given.

Appendix 2: Free food list   This lists foods which are very low in calories and therefore allowed freely in your new diet. Remember when planning your diet that there is a wide variety of fibre-rich vegetables and fruits to choose from in this appendix.

Appendix 3: 'Forbidden' food list   The foods in this list are those we generally advise diabetics to avoid. The appendix is included for two reasons: first, so that you can count the calories of the foods you are eating at present, and second, so that you can count the calories you have on exceptional occasions such as when you are ill (see page 32) or are going to take an unusual amount of exercise (see page 31).

It is clear from everything that we have said so far that we regard a restricted-carbohydrate diabetic diet as being unnecessary. We believe that in the light of present knowledge it is possible to recommend a wholesome alternative diet for diabetics which will result in improved blood sugar control and which may, in the long term, help to reduce the frequency of coronary heart disease. Such a diet is high in fibre-rich cereals and vegetables, low in fat and contains very little sugar. All diabetics need to ensure that they take the appropriate number of calories each day either to reach or to maintain ideal body weight. These principles of diet apply to both juvenile- and maturity-onset diabetics but there are enough differences in the planning of diets for people with the two types of diabetes to justify separate sections for each. Those in the former category can skip to page 24; while maturity-onset diabetics should read on.

The Oxford diet plan for diabetics not needing insulin

There are three golden rules for you to remember when following our diet plan:

1. Control your intake of calories;
2. Eat *more* high-fibre foods, and *less* fat and quickly absorbed sugar;
3. Have regular meals.

It is important for all diabetics to have some knowledge of the calorie values of foods. Ideally your diet should provide approximately the same number of calories each day. If your body weight is correct then you are probably consuming the right number of calories and all you will need to do is modify the kinds of food you are eating as explained below.

However, the majority of diabetics who do not need insulin are overweight. Most people can control their condition without any drug treatment provided they can reach their ideal body weight. Consequently for them the most important of the golden rules is controlling calories. Of course there will be those who will still need some form of pill treatment but they are in the minority and even they are likely to need a smaller dose of these drugs if they are able to get their weight down to normal.

Anyone who tells you that weight-reducing is easy has probably never tried to lose weight. Undoubtedly it is difficult, but the benefits in terms of feeling so much better in yourself, of avoiding antidiabetes pills, of improved physical appearance, of lower blood sugars and hopefully of a reduced frequency of diabetic complications make it worth the effort. And for those who are not overweight the diet is easier.

What is my ideal body weight?
We are often asked by our patients if they are overweight. It is sometimes said jokingly that the best way to find out is to take off most of your clothes and look at yourself in the mirror. This is not as silly as it sounds. Try it!

The first thing to do when beginning a weight-reducing diet

TABLE 1

Weight table for men of 25 years and over
(in indoor clothing)

Height ft in	(cm)	Small frame lb	kg	Medium frame lb	kg	Large frame lb	kg
5 1	(155)	112–120	(51–54)	118–129	(54–59)	126–141	(57–64)
5 2	(157)	115–123	(52–56)	121–133	(55–60)	129–144	(59–65)
5 3	(160)	118–126	(54–57)	124–136	(56–62)	132–148	(60–67)
5 4	(163)	121–129	(55–58)	127–139	(58–63)	135–152	(61–69)
5 5	(165)	124–133	(56–60)	130–143	(59–65)	138–156	(63–71)
5 6	(168)	128–137	(58–62)	134–147	(61–67)	142–161	(64–73)
5 7	(170)	132–141	(60–64)	138–152	(63–69)	147–166	(67–75)
5 8	(173)	136–145	(62–66)	142–156	(64–71)	151–170	(68–77)
5 9	(175)	140–150	(63–68)	146–160	(66–73)	155–174	(70–79)
5 10	(178)	144–154	(65–70)	150–165	(68–75)	159–179	(72–81)
5 11	(180)	148–158	(67–72)	154–170	(70–77)	164–184	(74–83)
6 0	(183)	152–162	(69–74)	158–175	(72–80)	168–189	(76–86)
6 1	(185)	156–167	(71–76)	162–180	(74–82)	173–194	(78–88)
6 2	(188)	160–171	(73–78)	167–185	(76–84)	178–199	(81–90)
6 3	(190)	164–175	(74–80)	172–190	(78–86)	182–204	(83–92)

Weight table for women aged 25 and over
(in indoor clothing)

(For women aged between 18 and 25 subtract 1 lb (½ kg) for each year under 25)

Height ft in	(cm)	Small frame lb	kg	Medium frame lb	kg	Large frame lb	kg
4 8	(142)	92–98	(42–44)	96–107	(44–49)	104–119	(47–54)
4 9	(145)	94–101	(43–46)	98–110	(45–50)	106–122	(48–55)
4 10	(147)	96–104	(44–47)	101–113	(46–51)	109–125	(49–57)
4 11	(150)	99–107	(45–48)	104–116	(47–53)	112–128	(51–58)
5 0	(152)	102–110	(46–50)	107–119	(48–54)	115–131	(52–59)
5 1	(155)	105–113	(48–51)	110–122	(50–55)	118–134	(53–60)
5 2	(157)	108–116	(49–53)	113–126	(51–57)	121–138	(55–63)
5 3	(160)	111–119	(50–54)	116–130	(53–59)	125–142	(57–64)
5 4	(163)	114–123	(52–56)	120–135	(54–61)	129–146	(58–66)
5 5	(165)	118–127	(53–58)	124–139	(56–63)	133–150	(60–68)
5 6	(168)	122–131	(55–59)	128–143	(58–65)	137–154	(62–70)
5 7	(170)	126–135	(57–61)	132–147	(60–67)	141–158	(64–72)
5 8	(173)	130–140	(59–63)	136–151	(62–69)	145–163	(66–74)
5 9	(175)	134–144	(61–65)	140–155	(63–70)	149–168	(68–76)
5 10	(178)	138–148	(63–67)	144–159	(65–72)	153–173	(69–78)

is work out a target weight to aim for. If you are one of those people who were lean until early adult life and then started to put on weight (quite a common sequence) then your ideal body weight in middle age is probably just a few pounds more than it was before you started to gain weight. If you are not yet middle-aged, or if you cannot recall a weight at which as a young adult you were lean you can consult the table on the previous page, which is a guide to ideal weights for people aged twenty-five or over, and decide with your doctor or dietitian what would be a reasonable weight to aim for.

If you have very mild diabetes and are on or close to your ideal weight
If you fit into this category your doctor may well feel that although paying attention to your diet is important you do not need to count your calories. In your diet you should avoid quickly absorbed sugar, lower your fat intake and eat more high-fibre foods. We suggest you use table 2 opposite as your guide. The foods in the left-hand column can be eaten regularly; those in the middle column should be taken in moderation; and you should avoid eating foods in the right-hand column altogether. We recommend that you use the recipes in Part II as often as possible since most of their ingredients fit into the category of food shown in the first column.

If you are slightly overweight and are not able to achieve your desired weight you have two options: make sure you have completely eliminated foods in the right-hand column and have even fewer of the foods in the middle column or start counting calories, as explained below.

If you are substantially overweight

Control the calories   To achieve weight loss it is necessary to count your calories, first in order to assess your present intake and second, to calculate your required intake in order to lose weight. The same principles apply regardless of whether you have just developed diabetes or have been diagnosed for many years and have never achieved ideal body weight or satisfactory control. Now is your chance! You should first determine your ideal weight as described above. Now comes the job of finding out how many calories you are taking in:

1. Write down in a notebook everything you eat and drink for two typical weekdays and for a typical Saturday or Sunday.
2. Use appendixes 1 and 3 to calculate the total number of calories (rounded to the nearest 10 calories) taken at each day's meals and snacks and then add them up to find the daily totals. It is easier if you have a doctor or dietitian

TABLE 2

FOODS TO EAT REGULARLY	FOODS TO BE TAKEN IN MODERATION	FOODS TO AVOID
Skimmed milk	Lean meat	**High sugar**
	Fish	Some types of alcohol
High fibre	Eggs	(see page 34)
Wholemeal bread	Cheese	Sugar/glucose
Wholemeal biscuits	Whole milk	Jam, marmalade and honey
e.g. crispbreads	Evaporated milk	Syrup and treacle
digestives	Plain ice cream	Mincemeat
Wholegrain breakfast	Yoghurt	Lemon curd
cereals	Margarine and butter	Chocolates and sweets
e.g. All-Bran	Cornflour	Cakes
Weetabix	Pastry (all types)	Sweet pastries and biscuits
Shredded Wheat	White bread	Sugar-coated breakfast
Porridge	Plain biscuits	cereals
Brown rice	e.g. cream crackers	Canned sweetened fruit
Wholemeal pasta	rich tea biscuits	Canned and other ready-
Wholemeal flour	Unsweetened breakfast	made or instant desserts
All vegetables	cereals e.g.	Sweetened desserts
especially:	Cornflakes	Mousse
peas, lentils	Rice Krispies	Sweetened fruit squash
baked beans	Special K	Sweetened drinks
dried beans e.g.	White pasta	
red kidney beans	Polished white rice	**High fat**
sweetcorn	Pudding cereals	Fried food
potatoes (eaten with	e.g. tapioca	Lard
their skin)	Unsweetened fruit juices	Suet
Fruit (with skin) fresh or	Malted milk drinks	Cream and cream cheese
stewed without sugar	Drinking chocolate	Cream soups and sauces
	Some types of alcohol	Dripping
Sugar-free	(see page 34)	Oils
Vegetable and clear soups	Dried fruit	Fat on meat and poultry
Tea or coffee	Coconut	Mayonnaise and
Sugar-free drinks	Nuts	French dressing
Oxo, Marmite, Bovril		Salad cream
Sugar-free sweeteners		Bought fish and meat/pâté
		Condensed milk

to help with this, and you may find it helpful, if some of the foods you eat are not in the appendixes, to buy a calorie-counter booklet that lists energy values for nearly every food and drink. Some are published by well-known slimmers' organizations and should be available in your local magazine or book shop, or public library.

3. Having calculated your total calories for each of the three days, simply add them together.

4. Divide this total by three to get your average daily calorie intake. Your new diet, on which you will lose weight if

you have done your sums correctly, should have about one-third fewer calories than you are having now. In other words, if your present average daily intake is 2,000 calories, to lose weight you should aim to have only 1,300 calories a day. It is especially important to consult your doctor before starting our diet if your reduced intake works out to be as low as 1,000 calories a day or less.

Some foods that contain very few calories are allowed freely on our diet and are listed in appendix 2. For all other foods, calories should be counted. Calorie values of the foods you should now be eating are given in appendix 1 and in each recipe in Part II. Many of the recipes are not only high in fibre, but low in calories, thus helping you to follow two of the golden rules. You will recall that fats have twice as many calories as carbohydrate and protein, and therefore the simplest way of reducing calories is to cut down on fatty foods. Check the high-fat section of table 2 to see which foods to avoid. Even though you are overweight, we recommend that you eat more high-fibre foods than you do at present. This means that to cut your total calories by one-third, you will need to reduce substantially your current fat intake.

Eat more high-fibre foods   While it is not necessary for you to count the carbohydrate values of the foods you eat as well as calories, to achieve good diabetic control your diet should be nutritious and high in fibre, and well balanced in other ways. The first thing to do is cut down on quickly-absorbed sugars; again, refer to table 2 to see the high-sugar foods to omit from your diet. Then, to make sure you are getting at least 50 per cent of your calories from fibre-rich carbohydrate, choose as many as you can both of the foods printed in **bold** type in appendix 1 and of the fruit and vegetables in appendix 2. You should also use the specially created recipes in Part II as often as possible (don't forget there are snacks as well as main courses); have at least two slices of wholemeal bread every day; have a substantial helping of cooked dried beans or a recipe containing them daily or at least several times a week.

Eat regular meals   If you are not taking antidiabetes pills it is not essential that your daily calories are distributed in precisely the same way every day. It is sensible, though, not to have most of your calorie allowance at one meal but rather to make sure that you have at least something to eat for breakfast, something to eat in the middle of the day and something to eat in the evening. If you are taking pills it is more important to have roughly the same number of calories and some carbohydrate at each meal to prevent blood sugar falling too low and producing a hypoglycaemic reaction. The most important consideration, however, is not to exceed your daily calorie allowance, set at one-third less than you are having at present.

Table 3 overleaf shows how someone currently taking in 2,000 calories a day might change to our high-fibre diet containing one-third less calories.

Once you have achieved your target weight you will need to find the number of calories which will enable you to maintain this. This will involve a certain amount of trial and error as you gradually increase your daily calorie intake until you are no longer taking off weight or putting it on; but once you have reached it life will take on a new dimension! You will now feel and look better, and be able to reduce the number of antidiabetes pills you are taking, or stop them altogether; but please remember that this must only be done in full consultation with your doctor.

Just because your new diet requires careful and precise planning within certain dietary restrictions this does not mean that from now on your meals will have to be unappetizing or dull. Far from it! The recipes and food lists have been designed to give you as much freedom as possible to work out a varied and interesting eating programme to suit your individual taste. On page 28 we have given some practical examples of how quite different meals can meet the same dietary requirements.

Will exercise affect my new diet?
Regular exercise should form part of your normal routine, and for normal exercise which you do every day like walking to work or riding your bicycle you do not need to eat extra food, as your planned diet should provide you with enough energy. If you want to take up a really strenuous activity like squash you may need to modify your daily intake, so you should first talk this over with your dietitian.

If you are not overweight but require large doses of anti-diabetes pills
We believe that if you fit into this category of diabetes you should be having a diet more like the one we recommend for insulin-requiring diabetics and we suggest that you follow the dietary advice given in the following section.

All other diabetics who don't need insulin can skip to the food hints section on page 32.

OVERLEAF: On the new diet calories have been reduced by one-third, fat intake more than halved, and starchy carbohydrate intake increased. All quickly absorbed sugar is avoided and the slowly absorbed carbohydrate from high-fibre foods increased so that total fibre intake is four times greater.

TABLE 3

AN EXAMPLE OF A DAY'S EATING FOR A MODERATELY OVERWEIGHT
LADY BEFORE SHE CHANGES TO HER DIABETIC DIET

DAILY:	*Cals/kJ*
This lady took about 380 ml/⅔ pt whole milk and about 10 g/⅓ oz butter	325/1,370

BREAKFAST:
2 cups of tea with milk and 5 g/1 tsp sugar in
each   40/160

SNACK:
50 g/1⅓ oz white bread roll with butter and
  20 g/⅔ oz Cheddar cheese
Coffee with milk and 5 g/1 tsp sugar   215/910

LUNCH:
100 g/3½ oz individual pork pie
150 g/6 oz fruit yoghurt
Coffee with milk and 5 g/1 tsp sugar   540/2,260

SNACK:
Doughnut
2 cups tea with milk and 5 g/1 tsp sugar in each   300/1,270

EVENING MEAL:
2 × 80 g/2¾ oz large fried sausages
Fried egg
100 g/3½ oz chips
100 g/3½ oz canned rice pudding
Coffee with milk and 5 g/1 tsp sugar   695/2,920

SNACK:
Chocolate biscuit
Coffee with 5 g/1 tsp sugar   150/630

TOTAL: 2,265 *Cals*   9,520 *kJ*

TABLE 3

A TYPICAL DAY'S EATING FOR THE SAME LADY ON THE OXFORD DIET PLAN
CALORIES ARE REDUCED BY ONE-THIRD

	Cals/kJ	Comments
DAILY: We suggest this lady should take about 380 ml/⅔ pt skimmed milk and 10 g/⅓ oz polyunsaturated margarine	200/840	Daily Whole milk replaced by skimmed milk to reduce fat intake. Fat allowance should include fat for cooking.
BREAKFAST: 60 g/2 oz Muesli (see page 108) with blackberries Milk from daily allowance Cup of tea/coffee with milk but no sugar	190/800	Breakfast Rushed cups of tea replaced by 5 minutes relaxation, a bowl of muesli and tea or coffee to drink. Remember no sugar but you can use artificial sweeteners if you wish.
SNACK: Cup of coffee with milk but no sugar Hazelnut crunchie biscuit (see page 98)	100/430	Mid-morning snack No hunger pangs because you have had breakfast, so one wholesome biscuit will suffice.
LUNCH: 2 × 50 g/1¾ oz Wholemeal roll (see page 93) With low-calorie liver pâté filling (see page 112) Slices of tomato and cucumber to accompany 100 g/3½ oz banana Tea or coffee with milk but no sugar	440/1,840	Lunch Pie high in fat is replaced by high-fibre wholemeal rolls with low-calorie pâté filling. Tomato and cucumber to give you vitamins and more fibre with very few calories. Sugary fruit yoghurt re- placed by banana.
SNACK: 2 cups of tea with milk but no sugar		Afternoon snack No need to eat at this time. If you must, have a crisp- bread or fresh fruit.
EVENING MEAL: Haricot bean and vegetable casserole (see page 63) 100 g/3½ oz potato boiled in skin Broccoli spears Sparkling fruit salad (see page 101) Tea or coffee with milk but no sugar	450/1,870	Evening meal Fatty meal high in calories replaced by satisfying casserole and potato. Fill up on free vegetables from appendix 2. Canned sugary pudding is replaced by a low-calorie dessert.
SNACK: Milky coffee (skimmed milk) with no sugar 2 crispbreads	60/250	Bedtime snack Coffee made with the rest of your skimmed milk and a couple of crispbreads to last through till the morning.

TOTAL: 1,440 *Cals* 6,030 *kJ*

The Oxford diet plan for diabetics needing insulin

As with diabetics who don't need insulin, there are three golden rules for you to remember when following our diet plan:

1. Control your intake of calories;
2. Eat *more* high-fibre foods, and *less* fat and avoid quickly absorbed sugar altogether;
3. Have regular meals: three main meals and up to three snacks each day.

This last rule is particularly important for you, and is discussed in detail later on.

If your diabetes has just been diagnosed

If your diabetes has just been diagnosed you may be admitted to hospital where your diet will be worked out with you by a dietitian. However, it is becoming more common these days, even when insulin is necessary, for diabetics to be started on treatment at home; and as far as diet is concerned there should be no problems, provided help is available from your dietitian, doctor or nurse.

Control the calories   First, it is necessary to count the calories you are at present having each day. We suggest you write down *everything* you eat and drink on two typical weekdays and a typical Saturday or Sunday. Then, together with your medical adviser, consult the calorie values in appendixes 1 and 3 and write down next to each food item on your list its calorie value (rounded to the nearest 10 calories). You may find it helpful, if some of the foods you eat are not in the appendixes, to buy a calorie-counter booklet that lists energy values for nearly every food and drink. Some are published by well-known slimmers' organizations and should be available in your local magazine or book shop, or public library. Add together all the values for each day and then calculate your average daily intake by dividing the days' combined total by three. If you are not overweight (see discussion on page 16) your new wholesome diabetic diet should contain approximately the same number of calories daily as you are having at present. If you are one of the few juvenile-onset diabetics who are overweight you should aim to reach your ideal body weight (see page 16) by reducing your present daily calorie intake by one-third. That is to say, if your daily average is now 2,000 calories, to lose weight you will need to cut down to 1,300 calories a day. There is an example on page 22 of how an overweight person on a diet containing around

2,000 calories a day changed to a daily intake of roughly 1,300 calories. This plan is useful for you only in so far as it shows how you might reduce your calorie consumption, for, as we are about to explain, for diabetics needing insulin, there are more considerations to be taken into account when altering your diet than are featured in the plan. Because cutting down on the food you eat will entail changes in your daily insulin requirements, weight reducing must be undertaken only with careful medical supervision.

When you have achieved your ideal body weight you can – again, in consultation with your doctor – gradually increase your daily calorie intake until you are no longer taking off or putting on weight.

Change to high-fibre carbohydrate foods   Once you have decided on your calorie intake, you should work out a sample day's menu using appendixes 1 and 2, and the recipes in Part II. We will work through an example later, but here first are the general principles. First, and most important, cut out all sugary foods (see table 2, page 19). Then, because we recommend that you have about 50 per cent or more of the calories at each meal and snack as fibre rich carbohydrate, find out the minimum amount of carbohydrate you should eat based on your calorie intake. Table 4 below is designed to do this for you. Decide which calorie intake is closest to your own and then read across to see how many carbohydrate units you require for the day. (1 carbohydrate unit equals 10 g carbohydrate.) Now chose your carbohydrate units from appendix 1 and the recipes in Part II. In appendix 1 high-carbohydrate foods are labelled with an asterisk and the quantity of food listed will provide 1 carbohydrate unit; the approximate calorie values for each item are also included. In Part II each recipe states how many carbohydrate units it contains and its calorie value. Once you have chosen your carbohydrate units, any spare calories you have left can be 'spent' on other foods.

To ensure that the carbohydrate you are eating is high in

TABLE 4

Daily calorie intake	Minimum number of carbohydrate units to provide about 50% calories from carbohydrate
3,000 (12,600 kJ)	35
2,700 (11,340 kJ)	33
2,500 (10,500 kJ)	31
2,200 (9,240 kJ)	27
2,000 (8,400 kJ)	25
1,700 (7,140 kJ)	21
1,500 (6,300 kJ)	18
1,200 (5,040 kJ)	15
1,000 (4,200 kJ)	12

fibre select high-fibre foods, which are printed in **bold** type, from appendix 1, eat plenty of vegetables and fruit from appendix 2, and use the recipes as often as you can (there are snacks as well as main courses). When planning your meals choose more beans, more wholemeal bread and wholegrain cereals than you have done in the past. To do this and still stick to your daily calorie allowance you will need to reduce your fat intake substantially (see list of fatty foods on page 19), and eat small portions of protein foods which come from animal and dairy sources – such as meat and cheese – because they are nearly always high in fat.

Your diet plan can be summarized thus:

1. Decide daily calorie intake;
2. Cut out sugary foods;
3. Use table 4 on the previous page to tell you how many carbohydrate units you need;
4. Use the recipes and appendix 1 to 'spend' all your carbohydrate units and calories, and to change to high-fibre foods;
5. Cut down on fatty foods;
6. Plan to have three meals and up to three snacks each day, each containing starchy high-fibre carbohydrate;
7. Remember foods in appendix 2 are very low in calories and are allowed freely. The vegetables and fruit are also high in fibre.

Now let's look at an example. Say you have decided that 1,700 calories per day is the correct intake for you; table 4 will tell you that you must choose a minimum of 21 carbohydrate units (more if you can without eating too many calories). You then turn to the recipes and food list in appendix 1 and choose your 21 or more carbohydrate units and additional calories for the day. Items in appendix 2 can be eaten as desired. Bearing in mind the points listed above, this is what you might choose:

		Carbohydrate units	Cals	kJ
DAILY:	380 ml/⅔ pt skimmed milk for tea/coffee and cereal	2	130	540
	15 g/½ oz margarine		110	460
BREAKFAST:	1 biscuit Shredded Wheat	2	80	340
	50 g/1¾ oz wholemeal bread (1 medium-size slice)	2	110	450
	Margarine and milk from daily allowance			
	Yeast extract (if desired)			
	Tea or coffee			
MID-MORNING SNACK:	Coffee or tea			
	One 15 g/½ oz oatcake	1	60	280

LUNCH:	Wholemeal spaghetti and			
	tomato sauce (see page 112)	6	340	1,430
	A good serving of mixed salad			
	Low-fat plain yoghurt with			
	chopped crispy apple or			
	any fresh fruit in season	2	120	500
AFTERNOON	Coffee or tea			
SNACK:	2 × 15 g/½ oz wholemeal			
	crispbreads	1	60	250
	with 60 g/2 oz Bean spread			
	(see page 107)		40	140
EVENING	Crispie-topped fish pie (see			
MEAL:	page 73)	4	360	1,510
	100 g/3½ oz jacket potato	2	90	360
	Casserole of frozen peas and			
	diced carrots sprinkled			
	with chopped fresh chives			
	Turkish apricot and orange			
	dessert (see page 99)	2	100	410
BEDTIME	Milky coffee using up daily			
SNACK:	milk allowance			
	2 Sweet and spicy wholemeal			
	biscuits (see page 96)	1	80	360
	TOTAL:		1,680	7,030

Here, the 25 carbohydrate units are well over the minimum of 21 and the calorie intake is extremely close to 1,700 (try to be within plus or minus 100 calories in your calculation for your total daily intake).

Eat regular meals   Your doctor should be able to prescribe your insulin on the basis of what he knows about your diabetes and the meal and snack pattern you have selected, though you might be asked to make minor adjustments. It is of the utmost importance that you select a distribution of meals that appeals to you because now comes the hardest aspect of all: it is essential once your insulin regime is established that you have the same number of carbohydrate units and more or less the same number of calories at each snack and at each meal every day, unless you are ill (see page 32) or are taking unusual amounts of exercise (see page 31). In other words, going by the example above, you should have around 250 calories and 4 carbohydrate units every day for breakfast, around 60 calories and 1 carbohydrate unit for your midmorning snack, and so on. Furthermore, the meals should be at the same time each day. It is most unlikely that you will ever achieve excellent control of your blood sugar unless you follow this advice.

However, being consistent with regard to timing, quantity and quality does not in any way mean that your diet must be dull and uninteresting. Quite the opposite. The whole idea of the recipes and food list in appendix 1 is that you can make up your daily allowance of calories and fibre-rich carbohydrate units in an extremely varied and appetizing way, adding as many foods as you like from appendix 2. To show you what we mean, look back to the evening meal in the example we have just given. Instead of making up the 8 carbohydrate units and 550 calories with Crispie-topped fish pie, jacket potato and casseroled vegetables followed by Turkish apricot and orange dessert you could have achieved the same result with either of the following meals.

EVENING MEAL:	Carbohydrate units	Cals/kJ
Dutch hot-pot (see page 63)	6	340/1,430
Crisply cooked spring greens		
Apple oatmeal crumble (see page 104)	2	150/640
with 60 g/2 oz Cream substitute II (see page 105)		40/170
TOTAL:	8	530/2,240

EVENING MEAL:		
Brown rice and tarragon soup (see page 39)	1	30/110
Small (25 g/¾ oz) slice toasted wholemeal bread		
(see page 93)	1	55/230
Spanish salad with potatoes (see page 45)	4	240/1,010
2 tbsp cooked red kidney beans	1	50/210
Crisp dessert apple	1	50/210
with a 30 g/1 oz sliver of Edam cheese		90/380
TOTAL:	8	515/2,150

Of course, you are not limited to just the meals we have shown here; the range of food combinations from the recipes and appendixes is big enough to cater for the most adventurous palate.

If you have had diabetes for some time
If you are not overweight your new diet should contain the same number of calories you are having now; if you are overweight, your new regime should contain one-third less than now (see discussion on page 18), and you will need to alter your insulin dose accordingly in consultation with your doctor.

Changing to our nutritious diet will be straightforward since you will almost certainly already be having three meals and two or three snacks containing the correct number of calories to match your present insulin intake. Note down everything you eat and drink on a typical day and calculate with your medical adviser the number of calories for each snack and meal using the calorie values in appendixes 1 and 3. Your new diet should contain the same number of calories on each occasion but substantially more fibre-rich carbohydrate, less fat and no sugar. To ensure at least 50 per cent of calories come from fibre-rich carbohydrate each day use the table on page 25 to see how many carbohydrate units you require for your particular calorie allowance. Then 'spend' them using plenty of high-fibre foods in appendix 1 (printed in **bold** type), generous amounts of the vegetables and fruits listed in appendix 2, and as many of our recipes as possible.

Unless your insulin regime is changed, each meal and snack should contain the same number of carbohydrate units and calories each day, and indeed all that has been said for newly-diagnosed diabetics applies to you; but probably you will already know most of this because the only new aspects will be the increase in high-fibre carbohydrate and decrease in fat.

Insulin, food and regular meals

It is sensible for everyone to eat regular meals, but this rule applies especially to diabetics on insulin. When the pancreas is functioning normally, insulin is produced as required in response to eating food. In juvenile-onset diabetes the body is dependent on insulin being available by injection at the times when food is taken. The oldest type of insulin was a kind of soluble or short-acting insulin and was given before each meal quite simply to cover that meal. This worked well but necessitated two or quite often three injections daily. With the modern types of insulin it is possible to control many diabetics well on one injection (which may consist of a mixture of more than one type of insulin) or two injections daily, usually given half an hour before meals. It is neither convenient nor desirable to change the dose of insulin each day because once the insulin dose has been decided there will be peak insulin activity at certain times of the day and these are the times when most carbohydrate must be absorbed from the food which has been eaten. If this rule is not followed it is impossible to achieve good diabetic control. Hypoglycaemic (low blood sugar) reactions will occur if food is not taken to cover times of peak insulin activity, and blood sugar levels will be unacceptably high if food is taken at times when insufficient insulin is available.

Some diabetics, however, are at present being inconvenienced in a way which we do not believe is necessary. What sometimes happens is that when someone is diagnosed as diabetic the doctor prescribes the number of meals and amounts of food at each to fit around the insulin dose that he or she has selected. Once the meal pattern has been started it must continue until the insulin dose is changed. For example, a common insulin regime is a twice daily mixture of a short- and intermediate-acting insulin. The times that these insulins will have their peak action is indicated in the diagram overleaf.

It can be seen that if this regime is recommended it is

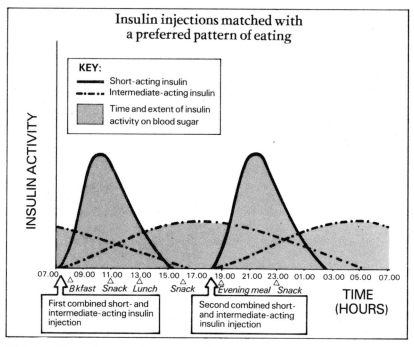

Insulin injections matched with a preferred pattern of eating

KEY:
— Short-acting insulin
—•—•• Intermediate-acting insulin
▨ Time and extent of insulin activity on blood sugar

INSULIN ACTIVITY

07.00 09.00 11.00 13.00 15.00 17.00 19.00 21.00 23.00 01.00 03.00 05.00 07.00

Bkfast Snack Lunch Snack Evening meal Snack

First combined short- and intermediate-acting insulin injection

Second combined short- and intermediate-acting insulin injection

TIME (HOURS)

This insulin regime would be suitable for someone who prefers a large breakfast and evening meal, and a small lunch. The peak periods of insulin activity cope with the raised blood sugar levels after the larger meals.

essential to have a fairly substantial breakfast, otherwise in the middle of the morning the blood sugar level will fall, resulting in a hypoglycaemic reaction. There are some people who do not like having more than a very small snack for breakfast and prefer having a bigger meal later in the day; and there is no reason why their insulin regime should not be modified so that they have only a very small amount of short-acting insulin in the morning, or none at all, rather than the amount which might be prescribed to allow for what the doctor considers an average breakfast.

Changing from a low-carbohydrate diet to our high starchy carbohydrate and fibre diet may need to be accompanied by a small reduction in insulin, and this must be discussed with your doctor. However, the main benefit to be gained from this diet is not so much the reduction of insulin as the improved blood sugar control which should result.

In summary, what we are saying is that to a considerable extent it is possible to tailor the way insulin is prescribed to fit *your* preferred eating pattern and that you should discuss this with your doctor. Of course it may be necessary to redistribute carbohydrate units slightly to achieve the best possible control and diabetics are often asked to do this. However, we do consider it of prime importance that you find an eating pattern which is acceptable to you because once this is established it is so important that you maintain a regular pattern.

Shift work Shift work often presents problems for the diabetic who needs insulin. For someone permanently on night shifts the problem may not be too great as you can simply reverse both the pattern of insulin injections and meals with some modification for days off work. When shifts alternate from day to day or even week to week it may be difficult to maintain good diabetic control. If your work follows this pattern, it is particularly important to work closely with your doctor to find the most successful food and insulin regime.

Special circumstances when you should change your diet

Exercise Regular exercise should form part of your normal routine, but remember that the more exercise you take the more energy in the form of calories from food you will need. For normal daily exercise like walking to work or riding your bicycle you do not need to eat extra food as your planned diet should provide you with enough energy. If you intend taking more than your usual daily exercise you will need to take more carbohydrate, as exercise uses up blood sugar.

For short bursts of strenuous physical activity – sprinting, swimming or rowing, for example – your body must have access to energy immediately so sugary foods such as chocolate bars or sweet soft drinks are needed. With this sort of exercise not only will you require food before the activity, but you may also need it afterwards.

For more prolonged, less strenuous exercise such as hill walking or cricket you should eat extra carbohydrate in the form of starch which releases energy more slowly into the bloodstream.

The amount of extra carbohydrate required for a given activity will vary from person to person. Initially we recommend you to take about 2–3 carbohydrate units before your activity and monitor the effect this has; you may find you need more food afterwards or even at half-time if you are playing an active team game. Below are some snack ideas, each containing about 2 carbohydrate units.

Snack suggestions for strenuous exercise
1 Mars bar *or* Milky Way (mini size)
4 squares chocolate *or* 3 toffees
1 chocolate-coated biscuit
1 glass of cola or other sweet drink
2 small bricks ice cream

Snack suggestions for more prolonged activity
2 plain digestive biscuits
1 large slice wholemeal bread with low-fat spread
1 bowl of wholegrain cereal with skimmed milk
1 small banana and a small (5¼ oz/150 g) carton plain yoghurt
1 crisp apple and 1 small (1½ oz/40 g) pack of nuts and raisins

When you are ill   At times when you catch influenza or other common illnesses, it is still necessary to balance your insulin with food. Even if you have no desire to eat, or feel nauseated, you still need to have *at least* your normal daily dose of insulin. In fact, frequently, you need more insulin when unwell even though you are eating less. Eating solid food may not be possible and so you may be forced to depart from your new diet and rely on sugary fluids to provide the necessary calories and carbohydrate. At times of illness it is important to ensure a continual supply of sugar to the body to prevent hypoglycaemia (low blood sugar). But it is not necessary to take the prescribed amount of carbohydrate at specific times of the day. If you are nauseated a few mouthfuls of sweetened liquid every fifteen to twenty minutes will satisfactorily maintain your blood sugar level. Here are some suggestions of food in light or liquid form, each providing about 2 carbohydrate units.

Snack suggestions for when you are ill
⅓ pint/190 ml milk + 2 heaped tsp Horlicks, Ovaltine or other
     malted milk powder
⅓ pint/190 ml milk + 1 tbsp/10 g rice or other dessert cereal
1 small (5¼ oz/150 g) carton fruit yoghurt
2 tbsp tinned fruit + 4 tbsp evaporated milk
small block of ice cream + 2 tbsp Ribena
⅓ pint/190 ml canned soup + 1 small slice bread and butter

Hints on food for all diabetics

Proprietary diabetic foods
Special diabetic foods are not a necessary part of any diabetic diet and are nearly always expensive. Fructose and sorbitol are the most commonly used sweeteners in these products. They do not contain glucose but do in fact contain the same number of calories as sugar itself. Thus foods such as diabetic jam, marmalade, chocolate and biscuits are just as fattening as their ordinary counterparts. Fructose is about one-and-a-half times as sweet as table sugar. Sorbitol is widely used as a sugar substitute and is about half as sweet as table sugar. Large amounts of sorbitol can cause diarrhoea. Intake of both these substances should be limited to a total of 50 g (just under 2 oz).

Synthetic calorie-free sweeteners

For most who require some form of sweetening agent saccharine, in tablet or liquid form, is the sweetener of choice. It has over 500 times the sweetening power of table sugar and is calorie-free. However, care should be taken if saccharine is used in cooking: wherever possible it should be added to food after it has been cooked, as it decomposes if heated and gives a very bitter taste. In some countries cyclamate sweeteners are available; these do not have such a bitter taste when heated. Powdered artificial sweeteners are best avoided as some contain sugar.

Unsweetened foods

There are now a number of products on the market which have no sweetening agents added. These include tinned fruits, jams and marmalades. They are more expensive than the sweetened products and once opened do not keep very well. However, as long as they are included in your day's calorie and carbohydrate allowance they are perfectly suitable, being lower in calories than the sweetened foods.

Diabetic drinks

The drinks listed below are all low in suger and suitable for diabetics. Many contain a trace of carbohydrate but not enough to be counted.

Boots diabetic cordials
Roses diabetic cordials
Energen One-Cal drinks
Lo-Cal drinks (Australia)
Tab, Fresca, Diet Pepsi
Weight-watchers drinks and cordials
PLJ (original and slightly sweetened)
Checkwate cordial
Schweppes Slimline drinks
Club, Hunts, and Canada Dry low-calorie drinks

Unsweetened fruit juices   These contain natural sugars and should be counted as part of your carbohydrate allowance. A small glass (4 fl oz/125 ml) of unsweetened orange, grapefruit, pineapple or apple juice gives about 1 carbohydrate unit (10 g carbohydrate). It is a good idea to drink fruit juice only when you are eating some other starchy carbohydrate food, especially those rich in fibre. The carbohydrate from drinks is quickly absorbed when they are drunk on their own, and this will be prevented by the other food to some extent.

Alcohol   Most alcoholic drinks contain carbohydrate, but it is better to consider this extra to your daily allowance of carbohydrate as the carbohydrate is quickly absorbed and doesn't have a lasting effect; but you must count the calorie contribution of alcoholic drinks. It is *not* a good idea to exchange the carbohydrate in alcohol for a meal or snack and it is better to drink after a meal than to have a drink before.

For diabetics alcohol has many effects ranging from a feeling of lightheadedness and well-being to nausea, coma or extreme illness. The more you drink, the more it affects you. The lightheaded feeling associated with alcohol can be similar to the symptoms of hypoglycaemia (low blood sugar) and it is easy to mistake one for the other. Alcohol also reduces the body's defence against low blood sugar, so it is better consumed in small quantities.

Alcoholic drinks to limit   Spirits such as whisky, brandy, gin, vodka and rum are carbohydrate-free but contain a lot of alcohol and are best limited.

Alcoholic drinks to avoid   Alcohol with a high sugar content such as sweet sherry and wine, port and liqueurs. Avoid also diabetic beer or lager. Compared with ordinary beers these are lower in carbohydrate but are more alcoholic, therefore it is better to have ordinary beer or lager.

In summary, then, remember the following points:

1. Drink in moderation; ½ pint/350 ml of ordinary beer or lager, or a glass of dry wine;
2. Count the calories but not the carbohydrate content when integrating alcoholic drinks into your diet plan;
3. Don't exchange alcoholic drinks for snacks or meals and don't miss out snacks while drinking;
4. Don't drink alcohol on its own; where possible drink with snacks or, best of all, at the end of meals.

PART II

The Recipes

INTRODUCTION

Weights and measures

The tablespoon measurement used throughout the book equals 15 ml and the teaspoon 5 ml; both are level unless otherwise stated. Calories (Cals) have been rounded off to the nearest 10, as have kilojoules (kJ). Carbohydrate has been rounded off to the nearest 10 g and is also given in units, each equalling 10 g. If below 5 g, the carbohydrate value is stated as negligible. Fibre, protein and fat values have been rounded to the nearest gram.

Ingredients

We recommend that you use the following ingredients in your cooking:

- Wholemeal (also called wholewheat) breads, flours and pastas; brown rice and pulses.
- When buying wholemeal flour, make sure it is 100% – that is, unrefined.
- Skimmed milk or reconstituted dried skimmed milk.
- Cheeses made from skimmed milk, such as cottage and curd cheese (provided they are labelled as low fat).
- Polyunsaturated margarines and low-fat spreads and polyunsaturated oils, such as corn, soya or sunflower.
- Fish and meat low in fat (with all visible fat trimmed from meat).
- Fresh fruit and vegetables with the skins left on, if possible. Frozen and canned may be substituted, but check that sugar has not been added.
- Herbs and spices – these are always a matter of personal preference and the amounts can be adjusted to suit individual tastes. The quantities given are usually for fresh herbs; frozen herbs are the best alternative, but if using dried herbs, use about ⅓ of the amount stated.
- Sugar-free liquid sweetener.

Cooking and preparation

- Grill, bake, steam or boil in place of frying.
- Use non-stick pans, casseroles and baking dishes to reduce cooking oil or fat to a minimum.
- When baking larger pieces of meat and some vegetables use roasting bags or foil covering to retain the juices and keep the food tender.
- Glaze pies with skimmed milk instead of egg and milk.
- Make sauces by blending the thickening agent with the liquid and bring to the boil, stirring, rather than by melting the fat, adding the thickener and making a roux.
- When making wholemeal pastry a good way of overcoming the problem of making holes in the dough when rolling it out is to roll it between sheets of polythene or greaseproof paper.
- In recipes which feature stock you can use stock cubes if you don't have home-made stock. Where the stock flavour is not specified, use whichever you like.
- All soups will keep for two days in a refrigerator.

Pulses

Many supermarkets now stock a wide variety of dried, frozen and canned pulses and the unusual types can be found in Oriental food shops, delicatessens and health-food stores.

Soaking   Wash thoroughly and soak in cold water overnight. Alternatively, place in a pan of cold water, bring to the boil and cook for 2–3 minutes. Remove from the heat, cover and leave to soak for one hour. The weight of the soaked beans is about double their dry weight. In the recipes, where the bean weights are expressed as: a certain amount, soaked, this is the weight before soaking – in other words, the dry weight. Where weights of cooked beans are given, the dry weight has been included in brackets, where appropriate.

Cooking   Put the beans in a large pan with plenty of water. Boil rapidly for 10 minutes. Cover and simmer gently until soft, stirring occasionally to ensure even cooking. The cooking time varies according to the type and even those of the same type can take different times, depending on their age and the amount being cooked. If you cook pulses frequently, you may consider it worth while buying a pressure-cooker as this reduces the cooking times.

up to 30 minutes (*10 minutes in pressure-cooker*):	aduki beans British field beans mung beans peas split peas

30 minutes to 1 hour (*15–20 minutes in pressure-cooker*):	black-eyed beans black beans barlotti beans cannellini beans flageolot beans Continental lentils ful madames lima beans
1 to 2 hours (*½–1 hour in pressure-cooker*):	broad beans butter beans chick peas haricot beans speckled Mexican beans red kidney beans
3 to 4 hours (*1–1½ hours in pressure-cooker*):	soya beans

Leave the seasoning until after cooking as the addition of salt, vinegar, lemon juice or tomatoes tends to toughen the skin and prevent cooking.

Brown rice.
There are three principal varieties of brown rice. Long grain e.g. Patna – the grains remain separate and fluff up when cooked. It is used to accompany savoury dishes or it may form part of the dish. Round or short grain – is used for making rice pudding as the grains are inclined to become sticky and clump together when cooked. Medium grain rice with rounded ends – varieties grown in Italy and Spain are used for making risotto and paella, but are difficult to find elsewhere. Substitute with long grain brown rice, if necessary.

Brown rice has more flavour than white rice, and has a higher vitamin and mineral content, although the B vitamin, Thiamin, needed by the body to utilise carbohydrate will be lost in the cooking water unless the correct proportions of rice to liquid are used. These are – 1 measure of rice to 2 measures of boiling water and 1 level teaspoonful of salt. If there are cooking instructions on the packet, follow them: some varieties of brown rice require more than twice the quantity of water to rice.

Cooking Bring the measured amount of water to the boil, add the rice (washed, if necessary) and salt, return to simmering point. Stir once, cover tightly and simmer steadily for about 40 minutes or until the grains are just tender.

Leave alone when cooking – if the lid is lifted, steam will escape and slow down the cooking time and, if stirred, the grains will break releasing the starch inside, making the rice sticky and lumpy.

If the water has not been completely absorbed, leave uncovered over the heat for a few minutes.

Cooked rice can then be gently fluffed up with a fork, or copy the Chinese and leave the rice tightly covered on the lowest possible heat (on an asbestos mat if possible) for 10 minutes. It is a great advantage to have a heavy pan for this.

Cooking in the oven   Use the same proportions of rice to water. Put the rice and salt in a casserole, stir in the boiling water and cook in the oven for approximately 1–1¼ hours at 180°C/350°F/gas 4.

Reheating   It is often convenient to cook a larger quantity than required – covered, it will keep in the refrigerator for a week. To reheat, place in a pan with a little water and put over a gentle heat, giving an occasional stir, or place in an ovenproof dish with a little water, cover tightly and heat in the oven for about 20 minutes.

Wholemeal pasta

The principal varieties of wholemeal pasta are:

- Spaghetti sticks and spaghetti rings
- Macaroni sticks and short-cut macaroni
- Lasagne – broad flat sheets which can be layered or stuffed
- Caramelle – medium-sized shells
- Tagliatelle (noodles) – long, flat ribbons, made with added egg.

They can be bought in supermarkets, country stores and health-food stores.

Wholemeal pasta is suitable to include in your diet as it is high in carbohydrate, low in fat and has a good fibre content. It has more flavour and a firmer texture than ordinary pasta.

Cooking   If there are cooking instructions on the packet it is wise to follow them. Allow plenty of boiling water to prevent the pasta sticking together: approximately 4 litres (6–8 pints) water for each 450 g/1 lb pasta. Slowly add the pasta to the boiling water so that the water does not go off the boil. Stir with a fork to ensure it does not stick together or to the pan, and cook steadily, uncovered, until just tender, but still firm. The cooking time will vary from approximately 8–18 minutes depending on the size and freshness of the pasta. Drain well.

SOUPS

LIGHT SOUPS

Wholemeal pasta soup

Serves 4
Each serving: 30 Cals/130 kJ, 10 g (1 unit) carbohydrate, 2 g fibre,
1 g protein, negligible fat

875 ml/32 fl oz stock
1 medium-sized carrot, diced
30 g/1 oz wholemeal pasta

½ tsp garlic salt
seasoning
1 tbsp chopped parsley

Bring the stock to the boil, add the carrot, pasta and seasoning
and simmer, covered, for 10–20 minutes (depending on type
of pasta) until the pasta is cooked. Add the parsley, adjust the
seasoning if necessary and serve.

Brown rice and tarragon soup

Serves 4
Each serving: 30 Cals/110 kJ, 10 g (1 unit) carbohydrate, 1 g fibre,
1 g protein, negligible fat

875 ml/32 fl oz chicken stock
30 g/2 tbsp brown rice
½ tsp celery salt
seasoning

2 tbsp diced green peppers
1 tbsp finely chopped tarragon
2 tbsp chopped parsley

Bring the stock to the boil, sprinkle in the rice and seasoning,
cover and simmer for 40 minutes. Add the peppers and
tarragon and cook for 5 minutes. Add the parsley, adjust the
seasoning if necessary and serve.

Mixed vegetable soup

Serves 4
Each serving: 60 Cals/270 kJ, 10 g (1 unit) carbohydrate, 3 g fibre,
3 g protein, 0 g fat

1 medium-sized carrot, diced
1 medium-sized onion, diced
125 g/4½ oz potato, diced
100 g/3½ oz swede, diced
garlic salt

pepper
750 ml/27 fl oz stock
¼ small cabbage, finely shredded
150 ml/5 fl oz skimmed milk
1 tbsp chopped parsley

Simmer the vegetables, except the cabbage, in seasoned stock for ½ hour, or until the vegetables are tender. Add the cabbage and continue cooking for 10 minutes. Add the milk, reheat and add the parsley. Adjust seasoning if necessary and serve.

Variations
Use other vegetables in season allowing approximately 500 g/ 18 oz vegetables to 750 ml/28 fl oz stock. When alternative vegetables are used, the carbohydrate content per serving of soup may be altered. Check in appendix 1 and adjust to allow for more carbohydrate if necessary.

MAIN COURSE SOUPS

Spanish Basque bean and cabbage soup

Serves 4, twice
Each serving: 170 Cals/730 kJ, 20 g (2 units) carbohydrate, 13 g fibre, 11 g protein, 4 g fat

30 ml/2 tbsp corn oil
2 medium-sized onions, sliced
2 cloves garlic, crushed
1 small white cabbage, shredded

300 g/10½ oz dried haricot beans, soaked (see page 36)
seasoning·
400 g/14 oz canned tomatoes
2 litres/3½ pts stock

Heat the oil in a large saucepan and brown the onions and garlic. Add the cabbage, beans, salt, pepper, tomatoes and stock and boil for 10 minutes, then lower the heat, cover and simmer for 3 hours. Taste and adjust seasoning, if necessary.

If a smoother soup is required, let soup cool, put through a blender and reheat.

Red bean soup

Serves 4, twice
Each serving: 170 Cals/700 kJ, 20 g (2 units) carbohydrate, 12 g fibre, 10 g protein, 4 g fat

30 ml/2 tbsp corn oil
2 medium-sized onions, chopped
2 medium-sized carrots, diced
other vegetables in season e.g.
  100 g/3½ oz swede
  1 small leek
  a few outer leaves of cabbage
300 g/10½ oz red kidney beans, soaked (see page 36)

400 g/14 oz canned tomatoes (or fresh tomatoes)
30 ml/2 tbsp tomato purée
2 litres/3½ pts stock
bouquet garni (thyme, parsley, marjoram and a bay leaf)
seasoning

Heat the oil in a large pan, add the beans and all vegetables, except the tomatoes. Cover and cook gently for about 15 minutes. Add the tomatoes, tomato purée, stock and *bouquet garni*, bring to the boil then simmer for approximately 2 hours. Season to taste and remove the *bouquet garni*.

This soup may be served as a broth or put through a liquidizer, but do not blend too finely; leave some small pieces of coloured vegetables visible.

For variety, other beans can be substituted for red kidney beans.

Scotch broth

Serves 4, twice
Each serving: 110 Cals/480 kJ, 20 g (2 units) carbohydrate, 6 g fibre, 8 g protein, 2 g fat

225 g/8 oz neck of mutton or leg of
   beef, trimmed of visible fat
60 g/2 oz barley, scalded
115 g/4 oz dried peas, soaked (see page
   36)
2 litres/3½ pts water
2 medium-sized carrots, diced

100 g/3½ oz swede, diced
60 g/2 oz parsnip, diced
quarter small green cabbage, shredded
1 small onion, chopped
seasoning
celery salt
4 tbsp chopped parsley

Simmer the meat, peas, barley and water in large covered saucepan, bring to the boil then simmer for 1 hour. Add the vegetables – except the cabbage – seasoning and parsley and continue simmering covered, for about ½ hour or until the vegetables are cooked. Add the cabbage and cook for 10 minutes. Skim off any fat. Remove the meat with a slatted spoon, cut up finely and return to the broth. Adjust seasoning, if necessary, and serve.

Minestrone with rice and beans

Serves 4, twice
Each serving: 260 Cals/1,070 kJ, 40 g (4 units) carbohydrate, 12 g fibre, 14 g protein, 6 g fat

1 large onion, chopped
1 medium-sized carrot, chopped
1 stick celery (or use celery salt),
   chopped
1 ham bone (an estimate of 60 g/2 oz
   lean ham included)
300 g/10½ oz red kidney beans, soaked
   (see page 36)

2 litres/3½ pts water
15 ml/1 tbsp corn oil
60 g/2 oz lean bacon, chopped
60 g/2 oz mortadella sausage (or other
   Continental sausage), chopped
200 g/7 oz brown rice
seasoning
4 tbsp chopped parsley

Reserve 2 tbsp of the onion and put the remainder in a large pan with the other vegetables, the ham bone, beans and water. Bring to the boil for 10 minutes, skim the surface then simmer for 1½ hours. Remove the ham bone, cool, remove and chop any pieces of meat. Fry gently in the oil with the bacon, sausage and remaining onion for 10–15 minutes. Add to the beans and vegetables and bring to the boil. Sprinkle in the rice and seasoning and cook for about 40–45 minutes until the rice is tender. Stir in the parsley and serve accompanied by wholemeal bread.

Italian vegetable soup

Serves 4, twice
Each serving: 240 Cals/1,010 kJ, 40 g (4 units) carbohydrate, 14 g fibre, 14 g protein, 2 g fat

225 g/8 oz haricot beans, soaked (see page 36)
1 medium-sized onion, chopped
2 cloves garlic, crushed
2 young leeks, chopped
2 sticks celery, sliced
2 medium-sized carrots, sliced
3 courgettes, sliced
400 g/14 oz canned tomatoes
375 g/13 oz potatoes, chopped with skin on
¼ small cabbage, finely shredded
100 g/3½ oz frozen or fresh peas
170 g/6 oz wholemeal pasta, e.g. spaghetti broken into short lengths
4 tsp fresh basil, marjoram, thyme, chopped (or 1–2 tsp dried mixed herbs)
seasoning
6 tbsp chopped parsley
30 g/1 oz Parmesan cheese, grated

Simmer the beans for 20–30 minutes in 2 litres/3½ pts water. Add the onion, garlic, leeks, celery and carrot and simmer for a further ½ hour. Add the courgettes, tomatoes and potatoes and continue simmering for ½ hour. Add the cabbage, peas, pasta, mixed herbs and seasonings and continue simmering for 20 minutes or until the pasta is tender. Just before serving stir in the parsley and sprinkle the cheese over the top.

Haricot bean soup

Serves 4, twice
Each serving: 170 Cals/710 kJ, 20 g (2 units) carbohydrate, 12 g fibre, 10 g protein, 4 g fat

340 g/12 oz dried haricot beans, soaked (see page 36)
1 ham bone, cracked
2 litres/3½ pts beef stock
bouquet garni *(bay leaf, parsley and 3 cloves in a muslin bag)*
seasoning
30 g/1 oz polyunsaturated margarine
2 medium-sized onions, chopped
2 sticks celery, chopped
2 medium-sized carrots, chopped
90 ml/6 tbsp dry sherry (optional)
1 lemon, thinly sliced

Place the beans in large saucepan with the ham bone and water, bring to the boil and skim the surface. Add the *bouquet garni*, salt and pepper. Lower the heat, cover with tight-fitting lid and simmer for about 2½ hours, until the beans are tender.

Meanwhile, melt the margarine and cook the vegetables over a low heat for 20–30 minutes. Add to the cooked beans and continue cooking for 30 minutes. Remove from the heat, skim off the scum and discard the ham bone and *bouquet garni*. Purée in a blender or pass completely through a sieve. Adjust seasoning if necessary and reheat. Stir in the sherry, if used, and pour into a warmed tureen. Top with the lemon slices.

SALADS

MAIN COURSE SALADS

Chicken and brown rice salad

Serves 4
Each serving: 240 Cals/1,020 kJ, 30 g (3 units) carbohydrate, 3 g fibre, 13 g protein, 7 g fat

150 g/5½ oz cooked chicken, diced
2 tbsp tinned red pimientos, chopped
100 g/4 tbsp corn kernels
120 g/4 oz oranges, or tangerines, peeled and chopped
400 g/14 oz cooked brown rice (see page 37) (130 g/4½ oz dry weight)

Dressing:
15 ml/1 tbsp oil
15 ml/1 tbsp liquid from tinned pimientos
15 ml/1 tbsp wine or tarragon vinegar
1 clove garlic, crushed
seasoning

Mix the salad ingredients together. Mix the dressing ingredients and combine with the salad. Chill for 1–2 hours.

Pasta and haricot bean salad

Serves 4
Each serving: 370 Cals/1,540 kJ, 60 g (6 units) carbohydrate, 18 g fibre, 17 g protein, 10 g fat

400 g/14 oz cooked haricot beans (200 g/7 oz dry weight)
200 g/7 oz cooked wholemeal macaroni rings (100 g/3½ oz dry weight)
1 tbsp finely chopped fresh tarragon
1 tbsp finely chopped parsley
1 tbsp finely chopped chives

Dressing:
30 ml/2 tbsp sunflower or corn oil
30 ml/2 tbsp wine vinegar
½ tsp prepared mustard
½ tsp garlic salt
pepper
sugar-free liquid sweetener to taste

Combine the beans, pasta and herbs. Mix the dressing ingredients together, pour over the salad and toss well. Transfer to serving dish and chill for 20–30 minutes before serving.

Mung bean and courgette salad See page 47

Serves 4
Each serving: 250 Cals/1,060 kJ, 40 g (4 units) carbohydrate, 21 g
fibre, 19 g protein, 4 g fat

15 ml/1 tbsp corn oil
2 medium-sized onions, chopped
1 clove garlic, crushed
30 ml/2 tbsp wine vinegar
45 ml/3 tbsp lemon juice
125 ml/4½ fl oz water
450 g/1 lb courgettes
2 stalks celery, sliced

3 medium-sized tomatoes, chopped
1 tbsp oregano
seasoning
680 g/1½ lb cooked mung beans (300 g/
    10½ oz dry weight)
3 tbsp chopped fresh parsley
2 tbsp chopped chives

Heat the oil in a non-stick pan and cook the onion and garlic gently for 10 minutes. Add the vinegar, lemon juice and water and simmer for 5 minutes. Wash, trim the ends and cut courgettes into 2-cm (¾-in) slices. Add the courgettes, celery, tomato, oregano and seasoning; cover and simmer for 15–20 minutes until the vegetables are just tender. Stir in the beans, cool, transfer to a shallow serving dish, sprinkle with the parsley and chives and serve.

Saffron rice salad

Serves 4–6
4 servings
Each serving: 190 Cals/820 kJ, 20 g (2 units) carbohydrate, 3 g
fibre, 15 g protein, 5 g fat
6 servings
Each serving: 130 Cals/540 kJ, 20 g (2 units) carbohydrate, 2 g
fibre, 10 g protein, 3 g fat

Dressing:
15 ml/1 tbsp sunflower or corn oil
15 ml/1 tbsp wine vinegar
15 ml/1 tbsp orange juice
4 tbsp chopped parsley
1 clove garlic, crushed
seasoning
½ tsp prepared mustard

Salad:
340 g/¾ lb brown rice cooked with a
    little saffron
200 g/7 oz cooked smoked haddock,
    flaked
Garnish:
4 medium-sized tomatoes, sliced with
    skin
6 black olives, stoned and halved

Mix the dressing ingredients and toss with the rice and fish. Garnish with the tomatoes and olives.

Spanish salad with potatoes See page 47

Serves 4
Each serving: 240 Cals/1,010 kJ, 40 g (4 units) carbohydrate, 7 g fibre, 13 g protein, 4 g fat

680 g/1½ lb new potatoes, boiled in their skins and diced
60 g/6 tbsp chopped mixed peppers
1 large Spanish onion, chopped
2 hard-boiled eggs, chopped
60 g/2 oz lean cooked ham, chopped
170 g/6 oz frozen or fresh peas

60 ml/4 tbsp Yoghurt and tomato dressing (see page 118)
1 clove garlic, crushed
4 large crisp lettuce leaves
2 tbsp chopped spring onions, including green parts

Mix together the salad ingredients. Add the garlic to the dressing and mix with the salad. Arrange the lettuce leaves on individual plates, spoon on the salad and sprinkle the spring onions over.

Salade Niçoise

Serves 4
Each serving: 260 Cals/1,080 kJ, 10 g (1 unit) carbohydrate, 4 g fibre, 14 g protein, 21 g fat

1 large crisp lettuce
100 g/3½ oz tuna fish, flaked
15 g/1 tbsp strained capers
60 g/2 oz stoned and halved black olives
1 large green pepper, sliced

½ large cucumber, sliced
4 large firm tomatoes, sliced
2 hard-boiled eggs, sliced
60 ml/4 tbsp French dressing (see page 118)
60 g/1 small can anchovy fillets

Tear the lettuce leaves in half and place in the bottom of a large salad bowl. Sprinkle the tuna fish over the lettuce with the capers and half the olives. Add the pepper, cucumber, tomatoes and eggs. Lightly toss with the French dressing. Garnish with the anchovy fillets and remaining olives.

Red bean salad

Serves 4
Each serving: 280 Cals/1,190 kJ, 40 g (4 units) carbohydrate, 23 g fibre, 20 g protein, 5 g fat

350 g/12½ oz red kidney beans, soaked (see page 36)
1 medium-sized onion, finely chopped
few crisp lettuce leaves, to accompany
Dressing:
15 ml/1 tbsp red wine vinegar
1 tsp salt

1 tsp French mustard
1 clove garlic, crushed
dash Tabasco sauce
pepper
15 ml/1 tbsp corn oil
1 medium-sized green pepper, finely chopped

Cook the beans (see page 36). While still warm toss with the onion in the salad dressing. When this mixture is cold add pepper, cover and leave in a cold place to marinate for 12 hours. Serve on crisp lettuce leaves.

Rice and aduki bean salad

Serves 4
Each serving: 430 Cals/1,820 kJ, 70 g (7 units) carbohydrate, 20 g **fibre,** 22 g protein, 9 g fat

200 g/7 oz cooked brown rice (70 g/
  2½ oz dry weight)
300 g/10½ oz cooked aduki beans
1 large green pepper, chopped
½ medium-sized cucumber, diced with
  skin on
3 stalks celery, chopped
6 spring onions, green and white parts,
  chopped

Dressing:
30 ml/2 tbsp corn or sunflower oil
30 ml/2 tbsp vinegar
1 clove garlic, crushed
½ tsp salt or celery salt
½ tsp dry mustard
½ tsp pepper
dash soy sauce
2 tbsp chopped parsley

Mix the salad ingredients together. Mix the dressing ingredients and toss well with the salad. Garnish with the parsley and serve immediately.

ACCOMPANIMENT SALADS

Brown rice and apricot salad

Serves 4
Each serving: 220 Cals/920 kJ, 30 g (3 units) carbohydrate, 8 g **fibre,** 3 g protein, 9 g fat

200 g/7 oz cooked long-grain brown
  rice (70 g/2½ oz dry weight)
60 g/2 oz raisins, chopped
85 g/3 oz dried apricots, chopped
4 spring onions, chopped
3 tbsp chopped parsley
Dressing:
30 ml/2 tbsp sunflower or corn oil

30 ml/2 tbsp lemon juice
30 ml/2 tbsp orange juice
10 g/1 tbsp walnuts, finely chopped
¼ tsp celery salt
¼ tsp garlic salt
pepper

Combine the salad ingredients. Whisk together the dressing ingredients and add to the salad. Leave for 20 minutes before serving.

Rice and aduki bean salad (*top*), Mung bean and courgette salad (*centre*, see page 44), Spanish salad with potatoes (see page 45).

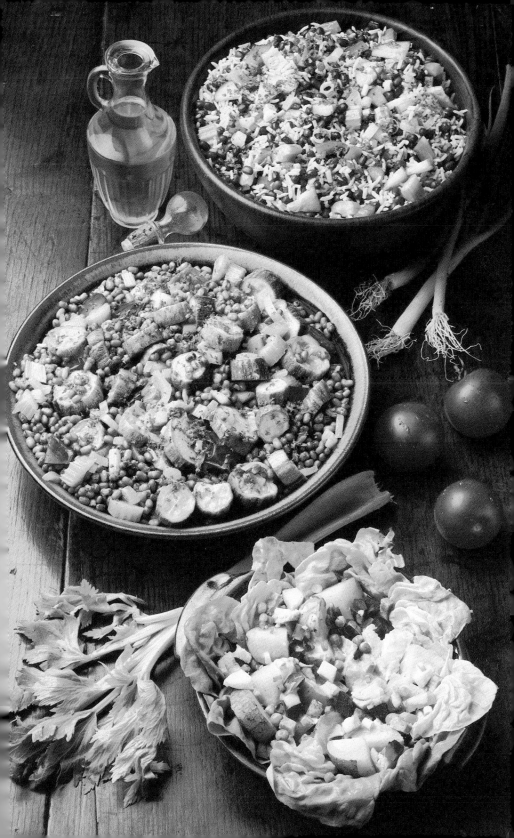

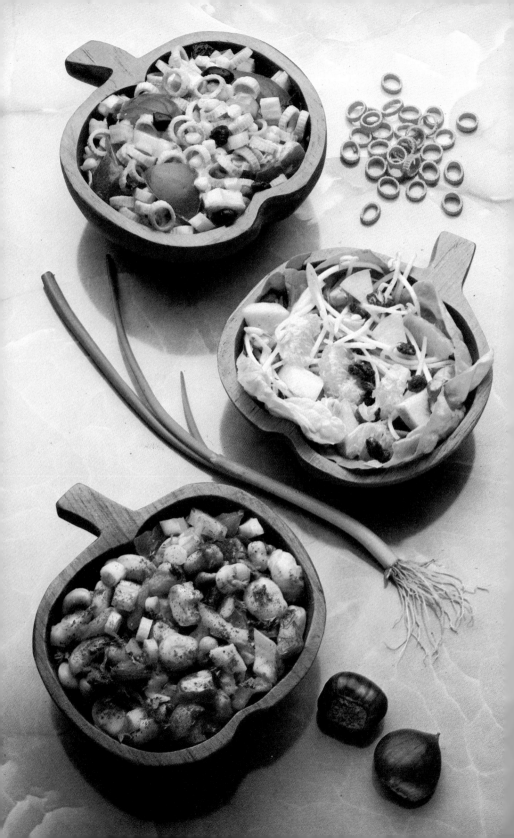

Beansprout salad

Serves 4–6
4 servings
**Each serving: 140 Cals/580 kJ, 20 g (2 units) carbohydrate, 7 g
fibre,** 5 g protein, 5 g fat
6 servings
Each serving: 90 Cals/380 kJ, 10 g (1 unit) carbohydrate, 5 g fibre,
3 g protein, 4 g fat

*200 g/7 oz green apples, cored and
diced*
*240 g/8½ oz oranges, skinned, sliced
and chopped*
200 g/7 oz beansprouts
30 g/1 oz sultanas, chopped

60 g/2 oz hazelnuts, chopped
seasoning
*45 ml/3 tbsp Lemon and garlic dressing
(see page 118)*
*2 bunches watercress or crisp lettuce
leaves*

Reserve some of the apple and orange and mix the remainder
with the beansprouts, sultanas, nuts and seasoning. Toss
lightly in the salad dressing. Arrange the watercress or lettuce
in a border on a salad plate and pile the salad in the centre,
decorating with the reserved orange and apple. Cover and
leave for ½ hour before serving.

Broad bean and chestnut salad

Serves 4
**Each serving: 170 Cals/710 kJ, 30 g (3 units) carbohydrate, 12 g
fibre,** 7 g protein, 2 g fat

200 g/7 oz cooked broad beans
*200 g/7 oz cooked and skinned chest-
nuts, finely chopped**
60 g/2 oz dried apricots, chopped
2 sticks celery, chopped
4 tbsp chopped parsley
15 g/2 tbsp natural bran flakes

Dressing:
150 ml/5 fl oz low-fat plain yoghurt
15 ml/1 tbsp lemon juice
¼ tsp celery salt
¼ tsp garlic salt
pepper and pinch cayenne pepper
*4 spring onions, green and white parts,
chopped*
paprika

Mix together the salad ingredients. Mix the dressing ingredients
and combine with salad. Chill for ½ hour. Serve with the spring
onions and paprika sprinkled on top.

---

*Tinned chestnuts without sugar, or reconstituted dried chestnuts may be used.

Spaghetti rings and tomato salad (*top*, see page 51), Beansprout salad
(*centre*), Broad bean and chestnut salad (*bottom*).

Carrot and celery salad

Serves 4
Each serving: 160 Cals/680 kJ, 20 g (2 units) carbohydrate, 13 g fibre, 9 g protein, 6 g fat

2 medium-sized carrots, coarsely grated
1 large stick celery, chopped
200 g/7 oz frozen peas
60 g/2 oz dried figs, finely chopped
4 tbsp chopped parsley
15 g/2 tbsp natural bran flakes
Dressing:
150 ml/5 fl oz low-fat plain yoghurt

30 ml/2 tbsp fresh orange juice
1 clove garlic, crushed
grated rind ½ orange
seasoning
Garnish:
1 bunch watercress or crisp lettuce leaves
40 g/4 tbsp flaked almonds, lightly toasted

Mix together the salad ingredients. Mix the dressing ingredients and combine with the salad. Chill for ½ hour. Serve on a bed of watercress (or lettuce) and sprinkle the almonds on top.

Cracked wheat salad

Serves 4
Each serving: 140 Cals/580 kJ, 20 g (2 units) carbohydrate, 5 g fibre, 5 g protein, 5 g fat

100 g/3½ oz cracked wheat
4 spring onions, chopped
4 tbsp chopped parsley
3 tbsp chopped mint
3 medium-sized tomatoes, chopped
Dressing:
15 ml/1 tbsp corn or sunflower oil

15 ml/1 tbsp lemon juice
seasoning
Garnish:
crisp lettuce leaves
¼ medium cucumber, sliced
10 black olives, stoned

Soak the cracked wheat in water for 15 minutes. Drain and squeeze dry. Add the remaining ingredients and mix well. Line a serving plate with lettuce. Pile the salad in the centre and garnish with the cucumber and olives.

Mixed green salad in orange and lemon dressing

Serves 4
Each serving: 90 Cals/370 kJ, 10 g (1 unit) carbohydrate, 4 g fibre, 3 g protein, 4 g fat

450 g/1 lb firm white cabbage (about ¼ large cabbage), finely shredded
1 medium-sized green pepper, finely shredded
1 tbsp finely sliced onion

small bunch young spring onions, sliced, using white and green parts
bunch mustard and cress or watercress, snipped with scissors
30 g/1 oz sultanas, finely chopped

Dressing:
15 ml/1 tbsp corn or sunflower oil   5 ml/1 tsp lemon juice
15 ml/1 tbsp wine vinegar   garlic salt
30 ml/2 tbsp orange juice   pepper

Mix all the vegetables and sultanas together. Beat salad
dressing ingredients together and add to salad, tossing well.
Leave for 15–20 minutes before serving.

Spaghetti rings and tomato salad
See page 48
Serves 4
Each serving: 190 Cals/780 kJ, 30 g (3 units) carbohydrate, 5 g
fibre, 9 g protein, 3 g fat

100 g/3½ oz wholemeal spaghetti   Dressing:
  rings   *150 ml/5 fl oz low-fat plain*
200 g/7 oz cooked corn kernels   *yoghurt*
4 medium-sized tomatoes, quartered *60 ml/4 tbsp tomato juice*
4 large sticks celery, sliced   *2 tsp chopped oregano*
6 black olives, stoned and quartered *dash Tabasco sauce*
2 tbsp chopped parsley   *seasoning*

Boil the spaghetti in salted water for 9–11 minutes. Drain and
rinse under cold running water. Mix with the corn, tomatoes
and celery. Mix together the ingredients for the dressing. Pour
over the spaghetti and toss well. Transfer to a salad bowl,
scatter olives and parsley over the top. Cover and chill for 20–
30 minutes before serving.

VEGETABLE DISHES

Oatmeal crunchy pie
Serves 4
Each serving: 400 Cals/1,700 kJ, 40 (4 units) carbohydrate, 6 g
fibre, 16 g protein, 24 g fat

Pastry: Filling:
70 g/2½ oz medium fine oatmeal   *2 large tomatoes, chopped*
115 g/4 oz wholemeal flour   *2 medium-sized onions, finely chopped*
salt   *100 g/3½ oz Edam cheese, grated*
70 g/2½ oz polyunsaturated margarine *15 g/½ oz Parmesan cheese, grated*
15 ml/1 tbsp (approx) cold water   *1 tbsp tomato purée*
                                      1 tbsp oregano
                                      seasoning

Heat the oven to 200°C/400°F/gas 6.

To make the pastry mix the oatmeal, flour and salt, rub in the margarine until the mixture resembles breadcrumbs, then mix with cold water to make a firm dough. Roll out two-thirds into a round to line the base of an 18-cm (7-in) flan tin and work the pastry up the side of the flan case with the fingers.

For the filling, mix the ingredients together and spoon into the oatmeal pastry case. Carefully roll out the remaining pastry and cover the pie. The pastry is extremely crumbly and great care is required. Fork the edges and prick the centre. Place on a baking tray and bake for one hour.

Marinated mushroom kebabs

Serves 4

Each serving: 70 Cals/290 kJ, negligible (0 units) carbohydrate, 3 g fibre, 4 g protein, 5 g fat

450 g/1 lb button mushrooms
150 ml/5 fl oz plain low-fat yoghurt
15 ml/1 tbsp corn or other oil
15 ml/1 tbsp lemon juice
1 tsp lemon rind
1 tbsp crushed bay leaf
1 tbsp thyme
1 clove garlic, crushed
seasoning
2 cartons mustard and cress or sprigs of
  watercress

Trim stalks from mushrooms. Put the yoghurt in large bowl, beat in the oil, lemon rind and juice and stir in the herbs, garlic and seasoning. Add the mushrooms and leave to marinate at room temperature for 2 hours, turning several times. Thread mushrooms on to kebab skewers and place under a hot grill for 4 minutes or until cooked. Serve on a bed of mustard and cress or watercress, spooning the remaining marinade over the kebabs.

Rotkohl (spiced red cabbage)

Serves 4–6

4 servings

Each serving: 70 Cals/310 kJ, 10 g (1 unit) carbohydrate, 7 g fibre, 3 g protein, 1 g fat

6 servings

Each serving: 50 Cals/200 kJ, 10 g (1 unit) carbohydrate, 5 g fibre, 2 g protein, 1 g fat

1 small red cabbage, trimmed and
  finely sliced
7 g/¼ oz polyunsaturated margarine
250 ml/9 fl oz cold water
2 small onions, chopped
4 cloves
1 bay leaf
2 tbsp dry wine
seasoning
200 g/7 oz cooking apple, cored and
  sliced

Blanch the cabbage in boiling water for 2 minutes and drain. Melt the margarine and toss in the cabbage for about 5 minutes. Add the water, onion, cloves, bay leaf, wine and seasoning and simmer for 20 minutes. Add the apple and simmer for 10 minutes. Remove the cloves and bay leaf and serve.

Broad beans with savory

Serves 4
Each serving: 180 Cals/770 kJ, 20 g (2 units) carbohydrate, 10 g **fibre,** 10 g protein, 9 g fat

30 ml/2 tbsp corn oil
1 medium-sized onion, chopped
1 clove garlic, crushed
1 tbsp chopped parsley
1 tsp chopped savory

½ tsp chopped lovage
900 g/2 lb broad beans
salt
nutmeg
140 ml/5 fl oz water

Heat the oil and cook the onion and garlic slowly for 10–15 minutes. Add the remaining ingredients, cover tightly and cook until tender. Drain the excess liquid and serve.

Baked stuffed potatoes with vegetables

Serves 4
Each serving: 550 Cals/2,320 kJ, 90 g (9 units) carbohydrate, 22 g **fibre,** 23 g protein, 13 g fat

1 kg/2¼ lb potatoes, scrubbed and pricked
60 g/2 oz brown rice
115 g/4 oz butter beans, soaked (see page 36)
1 clove garlic, crushed
30 ml/2 tbsp corn or sunflower oil
seasoning
85 g/3 oz Edam cheese, grated

2 large carrots, thinly sliced
1 large onion, thinly sliced
1 small green pepper, thinly sliced
½ medium-sized firm green cabbage, thinly sliced
225 g/8 oz fresh beansprouts
4 tomato rings
4 onion rings
a few parsley sprigs

Heat the oven to 200°C/400°F/gas 6.
Bake potatoes for 1–1¼ hours until tender. Cook the rice (see page 37) and the beans (see page 36). Mash the beans and add the garlic, 1 tbsp oil and seasoning. When potatoes are cooked, cut in half, scoop out centres and mash into bean mixture. Spoon into the potato skins, sprinkle on the cheese and return to the oven to brown.
Meanwhile heat the remaining oil and cook the carrots, onion, pepper and cabbage over moderate heat for 5 minutes, stirring occasionally. Add the beansprouts, cooked rice and seasonings and cook for 2 minutes. Serve with the potatoes garnished with the onion and tomato rings and parsley sprigs.

Vegetable flan au gratin

Serves 4
Each serving: 540 Cals/2,280 kJ, 60 g (6 units) carbohydrate, 14 g
fibre, 20 g protein, 27 g fat

Pastry:
200 g/7 oz wholemeal flour
100 g/3½ oz mashed potatoes
70 g/2½ oz polyunsaturated margarine
pinch salt
Filling:
2 medium-sized cooked carrots
2 medium-sized cooked onions
125 g/4½ oz cooked potato
200 g/7 oz frozen peas

250 ml/9 fl oz White sauce (see page
116)
2 tbsp dried mixed peppers
½ tsp ground mace
½ tsp celery salt
¼ tsp pepper
30 g/1 oz Parmesan cheese, grated
2 large bunches watercress or lettuce
leaves

Heat the oven to 200°C/400°F/gas 6.

To make the pastry mix together the flour and salt and rub
in the margarine until the mixture resembles fine breadcrumbs.
Knead with the mashed potato until a ball of stiff dough is
formed. Roll to required size between sheets of polythene or
greaseproof paper. Peel off top layer of covering, lift dough on
the bottom layer and invert to line a 23–25 cm (9–10 in) flan
dish and bake for 15 minutes.

Chop the carrot, onion and potato and add the peas. Mix the
mace and seasoning into the hot sauce, and add to the
vegetables. Pour into the cooked flan ring, sprinkle with the
cheese and brown under a hot grill. Serve hot or cold with the
watercress, or lettuce.

Pasta ratatouille

Serves 4
Each serving: 320 Cals/1,340 kJ, 40 g (4 units) carbohydrate, 10 g
fibre, 13 g protein, 11 g fat

200 g/7 oz short-cut wholemeal
macaroni
30 ml/2 tbsp corn oil
2 medium-sized onions, chopped
1 clove garlic, crushed
1 tbsp oregano
1 tbsp basil

4 medium-sized tomatoes, chopped
4 small courgettes, sliced
200 g/7 oz young broad beans
125 ml/4 fl oz chicken stock
seasoning
30 g/1 oz Parmesan cheese, grated

Heat the oven to 180°C/350°F/gas 4.

Boil the macaroni in salted water for 9–11 minutes and
drain.

Meanwhile, heat the oil and cook the onion and garlic slowly
until tender and golden. Stir in the herbs, tomatoes, courgettes,

beans, stock and seasoning and simmer for 5 minutes. Combine the pasta and vegetables, put in a baking dish, sprinkle cheese on the top, cover and cook for 30–35 minutes.

Okra Olympia

Serves 4–6
4 servings
Each serving: 130 Cals/550 kJ, 10 g (1 unit) carbohydrate, 10 g fibre, 5 g protein, 7 g fat
6 servings
Each serving: 90 Cals/360 kJ, 10 g (1 unit) carbohydrate, 5 g fibre, 3 g protein, 5 g fat

680 g/1½ lb okra, trimmed and sliced   *½ lemon, sliced*
(or frozen or canned)   *seasoning*
30 ml/2 tbsp corn oil   *1 tbsp oregano*
3 medium-sized onions, finely chopped   *¼ tsp dark brown sugar*
5 medium-sized tomatoes, chopped   *90 ml/6 tbsp water*

Blanch okra, if fresh, briefly in a pan of boiling, salted water and drain. Heat the oil and cook the onions gently for about 10 minutes. Add okra, if fresh, and cook for 5 minutes (omit this stage if using frozen or canned okra). Add the remaining ingredients, cover and simmer for 20 minutes. Season and serve accompanied by pieces of hot wholemeal toast.

Potatoes with onions

Serves 4
Each serving: 250 Cals/1,050 kJ, 60 g (6 units) carbohydrate, 7 g fibre, 7 g protein, negligible fat

4 medium-sized onions, thinly sliced   *½ tsp dried mixed herbs*
pepper   *1 beef stock cube*
1 kg/2¼ lb potatoes cut in 5-mm (¼-in) slices

Arrange the onion rings in the bottom of a fireproof casserole and sprinkle with a little pepper. Place the potato slices on top and sprinkle with a little pepper and the herbs. Dissolve the beef cube in water and add to the casserole to a depth of 2½ cm (1 in). Cover and simmer for 30–35 minutes until the vegetables are tender.

PULSES

Red bean flan with red cabbage salad

Serves 4–6
6 servings
Each serving (flan and salad): 330 Cals/1,400 kJ, 40 g (4 units)
carbohydrate, 17 g fibre, 23 g protein, 10 g fat

Pastry:
100 g/3½ oz wholemeal flour
20 g/2 tbsp soya flour
¼ tsp garlic salt
1 tbsp finely chopped marjoram (or
  mixed fresh herbs)
30 g/1 oz polyunsaturated margarine
15 ml/1 tbsp (approx) beaten egg,
  from eggs for filling below
Filling:
300 g/10½ oz red kidney beans, soaked
  (see page 36)
2 small eggs, beaten
140 ml/¼ pt skimmed milk
2 tbsp chopped parsley
½ tsp celery salt

½ tsp onion salt
pepper
10 g/3 tbsp wholemeal breadcrumbs
60 g/2 oz Edam-type cheese, grated
Salad:
340 g/12 oz red cabbage, finely
  shredded
90 ml/6 tbsp tarragon vinegar
seasoning
15 ml/1 tbsp lemon juice
150 ml/5 fl oz low-fat plain yoghurt
3 tbsp chives, chopped
60 g/2 oz cucumber, thinly sliced
  (with skin on)
60 g/2 oz radishes, sliced thinly

Cook and drain the beans (see page 36).
   Heat the oven to 200°C/400°F/gas 6.
   To make the pastry, mix the flours and garlic salt together
and rub in the margarine. Mix in the herbs and add approximately
15 ml/1 tbsp egg to make a stiff dough. Roll out thinly and line
a flan case and bake for 15 minutes until set.
   To make the filling, add the milk, parsley, salts and pepper
to the remaining beaten egg, then add the beans. Pour into the
flan case. Mix together the cheese and breadcrumbs and
sprinkle over the top. Return to the oven and cook for 30–40
minutes until firm and golden. Serve hot or cold.
   To make the salad, blanch the cabbage in boiling water for 2
minutes, place in colander and thoroughly rinse in cold water.
Marinate for 1–1½ hours in the vinegar seasoned with salt and
pepper, turning frequently. Remove and drain off excess
vinegar. Stir the lemon juice into the yoghurt, pour over the
cabbage and sprinkle on the chives. Garnish with the cucumber
and radishes and serve with the flan.

OPPOSITE: Lentil and split pea loaf (*top*, see page 72), Red bean flan
with red cabbage salad (*centre and bottom*).
OVERLEAF: Dutch hot-pot (see page 63).

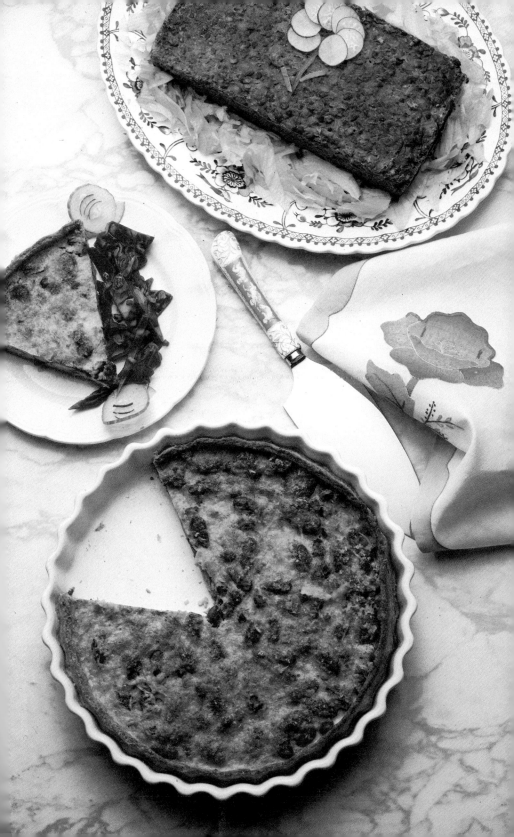

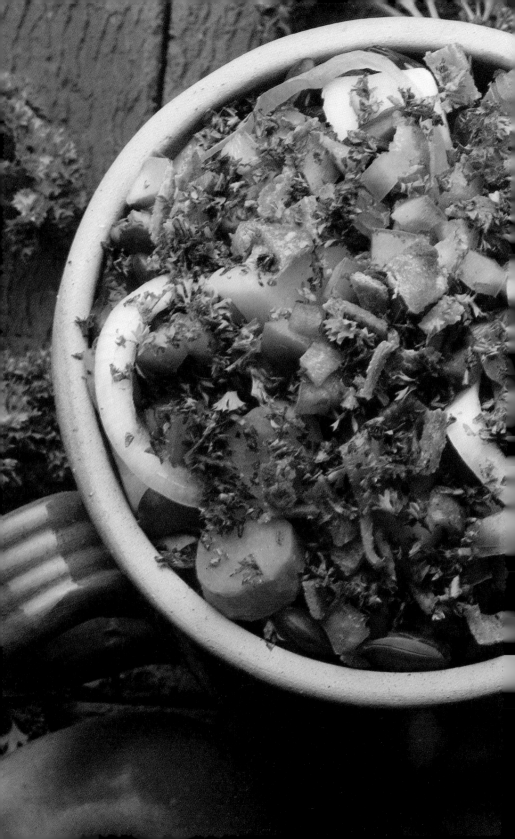

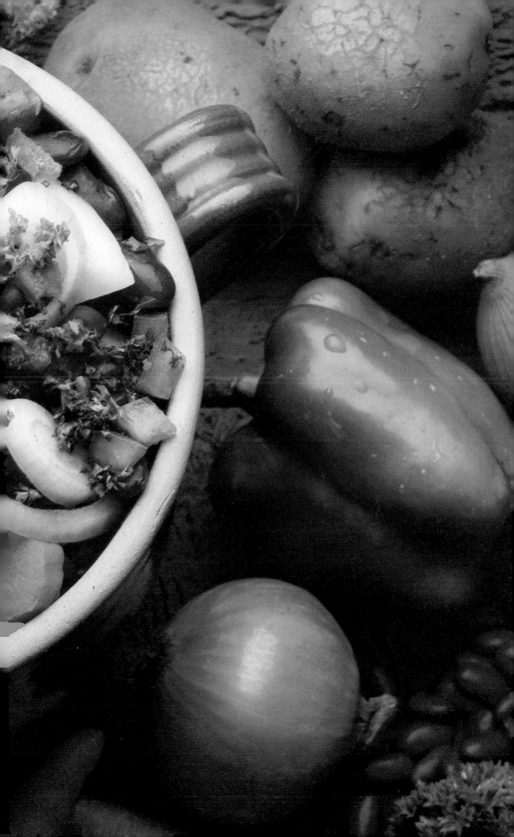

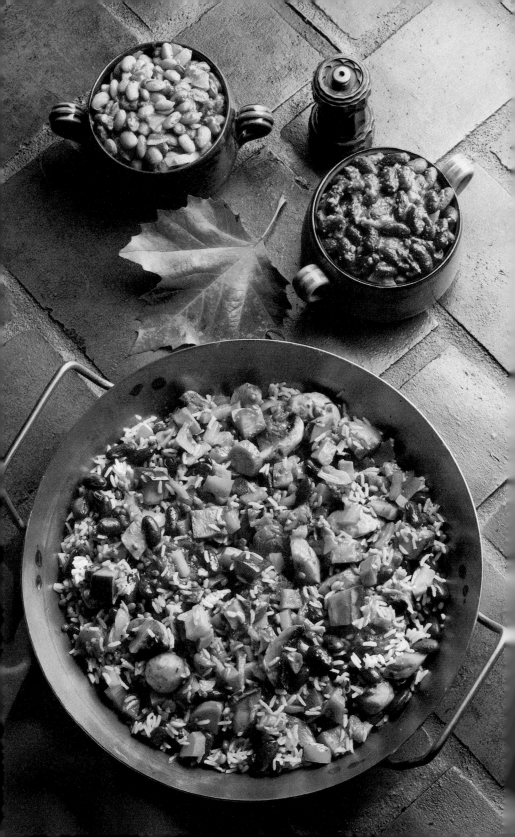

Chilli con carne

Serves 4
**Each serving: 530 Cals/2,240 kJ, 60 g (6 units) carbohydrate, 27 g
fibre,** 37 g protein, 16 g fat

30 ml/2 tbsp corn oil
2 medium-sized onions, chopped
1 clove garlic, crushed
170 g/6 oz lean minced meat
20 g/2 tbsp.wholemeal flour
25 ml/1½ tbsp tomato purée
250 ml/9 fl oz stock, hot

1–3 tsp chilli powder
2–3 drops Tabasco sauce (optional)
400 g/14 oz canned tomatoes
450 g/1 lb red kidney beans, soaked
(see page 36)
salt
1 medium-large green pepper, chopped

Heat the oil and gently fry onions and garlic for 5 minutes.
Toss the meat in flour, add to the onions and cook until
brown, stirring. Mix tomato purée with the hot stock and
gradually stir into the meat. Add the chilli powder, Tabasco
sauce, tomatoes and beans and boil for 10 minutes. Stir, cover
tightly and simmer gently for 1–1¼ hours until the beans are
cooked. 10 minutes before serving stir in salt and the green
pepper.

Alternatives
Use a mixture of meat and textured vegetable protein (TVP)
in place of all meat.
Instead of red kidney beans use haricot, butter or soya
beans. The cooking time should be adjusted (see respective
cooking times on page 37).

Vegetarian bean paella

Serves 4
**Each serving: 420 Cals/1,770 kJ, 70 g (7 units) carbohydrate, 20 g
fibre,** 16 g protein, 10 g fat

100 g/3½ oz red kidney beans, soaked
(see page 36)
60 g/2 oz mung beans, soaked (see
page 36)
225 g/8 oz long-grain brown rice
450 ml/¾ pt water
½ tsp turmeric (optional)
1 small aubergine, diced
30 ml/2 tbsp corn oil
1 Spanish onion, chopped

1 clove garlic, crushed
1 stick celery, chopped
1 medium-large green pepper, chopped
2 large carrots, diced
300 g/10½ oz canned tomatoes,
drained
115 g/4 oz fresh button mushrooms
seasoning
2 tbsp chopped parsley

Hot Mexican beans (*top*, see page 67), Chilli con carne (*centre*),
Vegetarian bean paella (*bottom*).

Cook the beans (see page 36). Meanwhile, cook the rice in the water with the turmeric, if used, and 1 tsp salt for 30 minutes (see page 37). Sprinkle salt over the aubergine, leave for 20 minutes then wipe dry.

Heat the oil and gently cook the onion and garlic for 5 minutes. Add the aubergine, celery, green pepper and carrot and cook slowly for 10 minutes stirring occasionally, then stir in the tomatoes and mushrooms and cook gently for 5 minutes. Gently mix the vegetables and beans into the rice, adjust the seasoning if necessary, then continue cooking gently for 15 minutes. Turn off the heat and keep the mixture warm for 10 minutes. Gently fork in the parsley and serve.

Country vegetable risotto　See page 69

Serves 4
Each serving: 440 Cals/1,850 kJ, 80 g (8 units) carbohydrate, 23 g fibre, 4 g protein, 1 g fat

200 g/7 oz haricot beans, soaked (see page 36)
15 ml/1 tbsp corn oil
1 medium-sized onion, chopped
1 clove garlic, crushed
2 large carrots, diced
140 g/5 oz swede, diced
½ tsp celery salt
¼ tsp pepper
1 tbsp marjoram or sage

750 ml/27 fl oz stock
200 g/7 oz short-grain brown rice
½ tsp turmeric (optional)
200 g/7 oz peas
3 tbsp chopped parsley
bunch of spring onions, green and white parts, sliced
30 g/1 oz Parmesan cheese, freshly grated

Cook the beans (see page 36). Heat the oil and fry the onion and garlic for a few minutes. Add the carrots and swede and continue to cook for 3–4 minutes, stirring occasionally. Sprinkle the seasoning and marjoram into the pan, cover with water and simmer until almost tender – about 20–25 minutes. Drain. Bring half the stock to the boil, sprinkle in the rice and turmeric, if used, stir and return to the boil. Lower the heat and cook gently adding more stock until the rice is almost tender (30–35 minutes) and the stock absorbed. Add the beans and the cooked vegetables and continue cooking for 10 minutes. Remove from the heat, adjust the seasoning, mix in half the parsley, pile on to a hot serving dish and garnish with the remaining parsley, spring onions and cheese. The consistency should be moist and creamy.

An alternative method is to boil the beans until half-cooked, then add the vegetables and rice. As different kinds of beans and brown rice vary in cooking time required, the first method ensures the beans are properly cooked. (The alternative cooking method produces a dish with a very low fat content.)

Alternatives
Many other vegetables may be used – potatoes diced with skin on, courgettes, broad beans, green beans, leeks and so on. The texture may not be quite perfect, but the distinctive flavour of mixed fresh vegetables is very good.

Haricot bean and vegetable casserole

Serves 4
Each serving: 300 Cals/1,240 kJ, 50 g (5 units) carbohydrate, 24 g fibre, 20 g protein, 5 g fat

*300 g/10½ oz haricot beans, soaked
(see page 36)*
15 ml/1 tbsp corn oil
1 large onion, finely chopped
1 clove garlic, crushed
2 outer stalks celery, finely chopped
2 medium-sized green peppers, sliced

2 medium-sized carrots, sliced
45 ml/3 tbsp tomato purée
1 tbsp oregano
4 tbsp chopped parsley
seasoning
250 ml/9 fl oz strong stock, hot
6 medium-sized tomatoes, halved

Cook the beans (see page 36). Heat the oil and gently cook the onion and garlic until golden brown. Stir in the celery, green pepper, carrots and beans and cook over a low heat for 10 minutes. Add the tomato purée, herbs, seasoning and stock and cook gently for 30 minutes. Place the tomatoes, cut side up, on top of the ingredients and cook for 15 minutes.
For variety, other types of beans may be used.

Dutch hot-pot   See pages 58–9

Serves 4
Each serving: 340 Cals/1,430 kJ, 60 g (6 units) carbohydrate, 20 g fibre, 23 g protein, 2 g fat

*225 g/8 oz red kidney beans, soaked
(see page 36)*
450 g/1 lb potatoes, cubed
2 medium-sized carrots, cubed
2 medium-sized onions, sliced
*150 g/5 oz cooking apple, cored and
sliced*

20 g/2 tbsp wholemeal flour
seasoning
*70 g/2½ oz lean bacon, grilled and
diced*
2 tbsp chopped green peppers
2 tbsp chopped parsley

Boil the beans rapidly for 10 minutes, lower the heat and simmer for another 20 minutes. Add the vegetables, make up the water to about 540 ml/1 pt and cook, tightly covered, for 30–40 minutes until the vegetables are tender but not soft. Blend the flour with a little cold water, stir in a little of the boiling vegetable liquid then stir into the vegetables and adjust seasoning, if necessary. Sprinkle the bacon and peppers over the top, then sprinkle on the chopped parsley and serve hot.

Although traditionally bacon is served separately, the flavour is improved when this is stirred in along with chopped parsley and other favourite herbs ¼ hour before serving. Garnish with more parsley and peppers.

Kidney bean risotto

Serves 6
Each serving: 370 Cals/1,550 kJ, 60 g (6 units) carbohydrate, 11 g fibre, 15 g protein, 7 g fat

15 ml/1 tbsp corn oil
2 shallots or small onions, finely chopped
2 cloves garlic, crushed
1 medium-sized carrot, diced
2 courgettes, diced
2 large sticks celery, diced
400 g/14 oz long-grain brown rice

1 litre/1¾ pts boiling stock
seasoning
300 g/10½ oz cooked red kidney beans (150 g/5 oz dry weight)
60 g/2 oz grilled lean bacon, diced
30 g/1 oz Parmesan cheese, grated

Heat the oil, add the shallots, or onions, and garlic and cook gently for 5 minutes. Stir in the carrots, courgettes and celery. Lower the heat, cover and shake the pan well and allow vegetables to cook in their own juice for 5 minutes. Stir in the rice and cook for 5 minutes, shaking occasionally. Add the boiling stock and seasonings, lower the heat and cook gently for about 40 minutes adding more stock if required. Stir occasionally. Add the beans and bacon and cook gently for about 10 minutes until the beans are hot and the rice is tender. Sprinkle the cheese over the top and serve.

Chick pea and leek quiche

Serves 4–6
4 servings
Each serving: 530 Cals/2,230kJ, 60 g (6 units) carbohydrate, 12 g fibre, 25 g protein, 23 g fat
6 servings
Each serving: 350 Cals/1,490 kJ, 40 g (4 units) carbohydrate, 8 g fibre, 17 g protein, 15 g fat

Pastry:
200 g/7 oz wholemeal flour
100 g/3½ oz cooked mashed potatoes
70 g/2½ oz polyunsaturated margarine
¼ tsp dry mustard
¼ tsp garlic salt
¼ tsp celery salt
Filling:
4 young leeks, sliced

1 clove garlic, crushed
250 ml/9 fl oz skimmed milk
2 small eggs
255 g/9 oz cooked chick peas
100 g/3½ oz skimmed-milk cheese
1 tsp onion salt
pepper
small bunch spring onions, chopped
30 g/1 oz Parmesan cheese, grated

Set the oven to 200°C/400°F/gas 6.

To make the pastry, mix salts and mustard with the flour and continue as for Vegetable flan au gratin on page 54. Line a 20–25 cm (9–10 in) flan dish, prick the bottom and bake for 15 minutes. Remove from the oven and reset the heat to 180°C/350°F/gas 4.

Meanwhile, heat the milk and simmer the leeks for 5 minutes. Beat together the eggs, cheese and seasonings. Add the chick peas, leeks and milk. Pour into the flan case, sprinkle the top with the spring onions and then the cheese. Bake for 50–55 minutes until filling is set. Serve hot or cold.

New England succotash

Serves 4

Each serving: 470 Cals/1,970 kJ, 70 g (7 units) carbohydrate, 26 g fibre, 24 g protein, 10 g fat

400 g/14 oz butter beans, soaked (see page 36)
15 ml/1 tbsp cooking oil
1 clove garlic, crushed
400 g/14 oz corn kernels
1 small red pepper, diced
seasoning
250 ml/9 fl oz Tomato sauce I (see page 117)

Cook the beans (see page 36). Heat the oil in large pan and cook the garlic and red pepper gently for 5 minutes. Add the beans, corn and seasonings. Mix thoroughly, cover and heat through for 10–15 minutes, giving an occasional shake. Serve with the tomato sauce.

Cannellini bean goulash

Serves 4

Each serving: 390 Cals/1,640 kJ, 40 g (4 units) carbohydrate, 17 g fibre, 18 g protein, 16 g fat

225 g/8 oz cannellini beans, soaked (see page 36)
60 ml/4 tbsp corn oil
2 large onions, sliced
2 medium-large green peppers, sliced
1 clove garlic, crushed
800 g/28 oz canned tomatoes
60 ml/4 tbsp tomato purée
4 tsp paprika
seasoning
150 ml/5 fl oz low-fat plain yoghurt

Cook the beans (see page 36). Heat the oil and gently cook the onions for 10–15 minutes, then add the green pepper and cook for 5 minutes. Stir in the remaining ingredients, except the yoghurt, bring to the boil and simmer for 15 minutes until the liquid has slightly reduced. Just before serving, stir in the yoghurt.

Haricot beans with bacon and tomatoes

Serves 4

Each serving: 560 Cals/2,350 kJ, 60 g (6 units) carbohydrate, 32 g fibre, 38 g protein, 16 g fat

450 g/1 lb haricot beans, soaked (see
*   page 36)*
15 g/½ oz polyunsaturated margarine
4 shallots or small onions, chopped
1 clove garlic, crushed
6 medium-sized tomatoes, chopped
seasoning

250 ml/10 fl oz cider or white wine
140 g/5 oz lean bacon, grilled and
*   diced*
2 tbsp chervil
60 g/2 oz wholemeal breadcrumbs
15 ml/1 tbsp corn oil

Cook the beans (see page 36). Melt the margarine and gently cook the onion and garlic until soft. Stir in the tomatoes, seasoning, cider (or wine) and beans and bring to simmering point and heat for 10–15 minutes. Stir in the bacon and chervil. Transfer to a fairly shallow heat-proof dish, spread the top with crumbs and sprinkle with drops of oil. Put under a hot grill until the top is crisp.

Serving suggestions
Depending on appetite this dish can be served as a snack by itself or used as a supper dish when hungry calorie-counters may serve crisp green vegetables with it.
    Diabetics in the higher calorie range could eat it accompanied by boiled brown rice.

Casserole of aduki beans

Serves 4

Each serving: 340 Cals/1,450 kJ, 60 g (6 units) carbohydrate, 22 g fibre, 16 g protein, 5 g fat

15 ml/1 tbsp corn oil
2 medium-sized onions, chopped
2 medium-sized carrots, diced
1 clove garlic, crushed
200 g/7 oz aduki beans, soaked (see
*   page 36)*

200 g/7 oz long-grain brown rice,
*   washed*
1 tbsp basil
1 litre/1¾ pts stock
115 g/4 oz mushrooms, sliced
15 ml/1 tbsp miso or soy sauce
salt

Heat the oil in a large saucepan and lightly brown the onions. Stir in the carrots and garlic and cook slowly with the lid on for 5 minutes. Mix in the beans, rice and basil. Add the stock and bring to the boil, stirring occasionally. Boil for 10 minutes then lower the heat and simmer for 40 minutes or until beans and rice are tender. Add the mushrooms, miso or soy sauce and salt. Return to simmering and cook for 5 minutes.

Baked bean lasagne

Serves 4–6
4 servings
Each serving: 490 Cals/2,060 kJ, 80 g (8 units) carbohydrate, 18 g fibre, 24 g protein, 13 g fat
6 servings
Each serving: 330 Cals/1,380 kJ, 50 g (5 units) carbohydrate, 13 g fibre, 16 g protein, 9 g fat

225 g/8 oz wholemeal lasagne
450 g/1 lb canned baked beans
45 ml/3 tbsp tomato ketchup
1 large Spanish onion, chopped
2 cloves garlic, crushed
1 large carrot, coarsely grated
200 g/7 oz canned tomatoes
salt

30 g/1 oz Parmesan cheese, grated
Sauce:
60 g/6 tbsp wholemeal flour
500 ml/18 fl oz skimmed milk
250 ml/9 fl oz water from cooked
vegetables
40 g/1¼ oz polyunsaturated margarine
seasoning

Heat the oven to 190°C/375°F/gas 5.

Cook·the lasagne in boiling salted water until half-cooked. Drain carefully.

Mix the beans and ketchup. Place the onion, garlic, carrot and tomatoes in a saucepan with a little salt, add just enough boiling water to cover, and cook gently till tender. Drain and reserve the cooking liquid.

To make the sauce, blend the flour with a little of the milk. Bring the remaining milk and the water to the boil and gradually stir into the flour. Return to the pan, add the margarine, oregano and seasoning and cook gently for a few minutes. Put a layer of the vegetables in a non-stick casserole or baking tin then a layer of lasagne, then a layer of beans, and then a layer of sauce. Repeat these layers finishing with a layer of sauce. Sprinkle the cheese on top* and bake for 35–40 minutes.

Hot Mexican beans   See page 60

Serves 4
Each serving: 210 Cals/890 kJ, 30 g (3 units) carbohydrate, 16 g fibre, 14 g protein, 5 g fat

15 ml/1 tbsp corn oil
225 g/8 oz speckled Mexican beans,
  soaked (see page 36)
2 medium-sized onions, chopped
1 clove garlic, crushed

6 medium-sized tomatoes
¼ tsp chilli powder
few drops Tabasco sauce
1½ tbsp oregano
seasoning

---

* This dish can be prepared in advance to this stage, covered and stored in the refrigerator, but allow 40–45 minutes for the final cooking.

Cook the beans (see page 36). Heat the oil and cook the onion and garlic slowly for 10 minutes. Stir in the remaining ingredients. Add the chilli powder very carefully – less than ¼ tsp is sufficient for many people – bring to simmering point, stir in the beans and simmer, covered, for 20 minutes.

Bean pie

Serves 4

Each serving: 520 Cals/2,190 kJ, 90 g (9 units) carbohydrate, 33 g fibre, 33 g protein, 6 g fat

225 g/½ lb red kidney beans, soaked (see page 36)
225 g/½ lb black-eyed beans, soaked (see page 36)
1 medium-sized onion, chopped
115 g/4 oz mushrooms, sliced
1 medium-sized green pepper, chopped
1 medium-sized red pepper, chopped
400 g/14 oz canned tomatoes

1 tbsp oregano or mixed herbs
seasoning
chicken stock (see method)
Topping:
680 g/1½ lb mashed potatoes mixed with
60 ml/4 tbsp skimmed milk
60 g/2 oz Edam-type cheese, grated

Heat the oven to 200°C/400°F/gas 6.

Boil the beans gently together for ½ hour. Place the beans and vegetables, except the mashed potatoes, in layers in a strong stoneware pot or casserole, sprinkling a little seasoning and herbs between the layers. Add sufficient stock to come about level with the bean mixture. Cover with the mashed potato and sprinkle with the cheese. Bake for 40–45 minutes until brown.

Lentil bake

Serves 4

Each serving: 350 Cals/1,470 kJ, 50 g (5 units) carbohydrate, 15 g fibre, 25 g protein, 8 g fat

15 ml/1 tbsp corn oil
2 shallots or small onions, chopped
300 g/10½ oz red lentils
4 medium-sized tomatoes, chopped
boiling water (see method)
1 bay leaf

½ tsp prepared mustard
60 g/2 oz Edam-type cheese, grated
10 g/3 tbsp wholemeal breadcrumbs
900 g/2 lb celery, chopped
2 tbsp chopped parsley

Bean pie (*above*), Country vegetable risotto (*below*, see page 62).

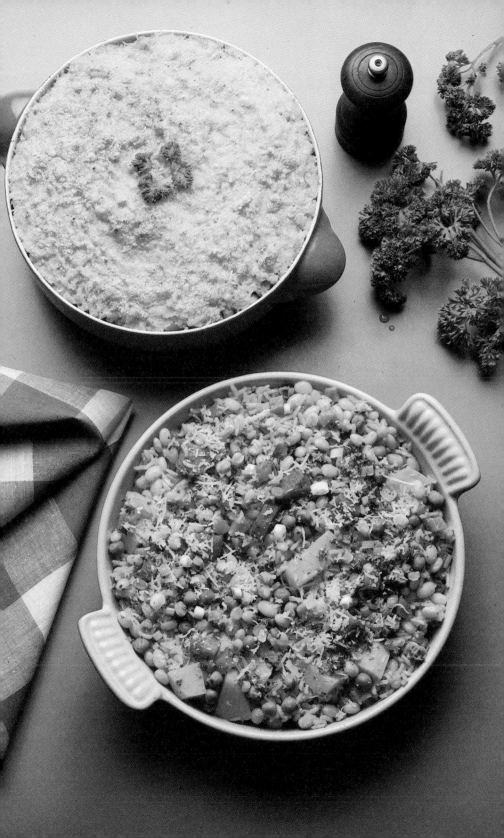

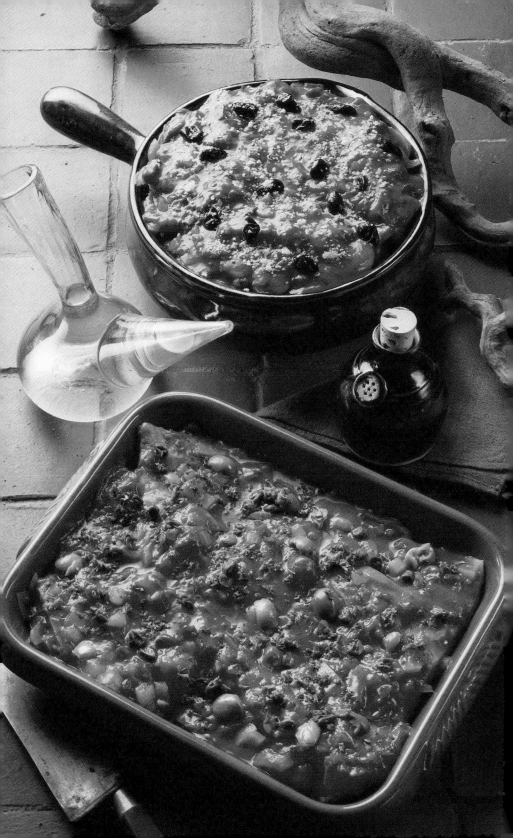

Heat the oil and gently cook the shallots or onions until beginning to soften. Add the lentils, increase heat and cook, stirring, for 5 minutes. Stir in the tomatoes and cook over a low heat for a few minutes. Just cover with boiling water, stir and continue to cook over a gentle heat for about 20 minutes until all the water has been absorbed.

Heat the oven to 200°C/400°F/gas 6.

Remove the pan from the heat, mix in the bay leaf, seasonings and cheese, retaining 3 tbsp for the top. Turn into a non-stick baking dish and sprinkle the breadcrumbs and remaining cheese over the top. Bake for 30–40 minutes. Remove the bay leaf.

Meanwhile, cook the celery. Sprinkle the parsley over and serve with the lentils.

Vegetarian lentil and cheese pie

Serves 4

Each serving: 560 Cals/2,350 kJ, 80 g (8 units) carbohydrate, 15 g fibre, 27 g protein, 17 g fat

200 g/7 oz brown lentils
115 g/4 oz yellow split peas
30 ml/2 tbsp corn oil
2 medium-sized onions, chopped
4 sticks celery, finely chopped
2 medium-sized carrots, coarsely grated
1 small green pepper, chopped
1 clove garlic, crushed
½ tsp dried mixed herbs
¼ tsp cayenne pepper

seasoning
4 medium-sized tomatoes, sliced
Topping:
1 tbsp chopped onion retained from
above
570 g/1¼ lb mashed potatoes
60 g/2 oz Cheddar cheese, grated
15 g/½ oz polyunsaturated margarine
60 ml/4 tbsp skimmed milk
¼ tsp grated nutmeg

Cook the lentils for 15 minutes, then add the peas and continue cooking for 30 minutes or until both are soft.

Meanwhile, heat the oil and cook the onion gently for 5 minutes (retain 1 tbsp for the topping). Stir in the rest of the vegetables, lower the heat and cook slowly for 15–20 minutes.

Heat the oven to 200°C/400°F/gas 6.

Drain the lentil and pea mixture and mash lightly. Stir in the vegetables, herbs and seasonings. Spoon into a large pie dish and place the sliced tomatoes on top.

To make the topping, add the sautéed onion, 3 tbsp milk (retaining a little to brush on the top), cheese and seasonings to the mashed potato and mix well. Spread over the tomatoes and brush over with the remaining milk. Bake for about 30 minutes.

Tuna Provençal (*above*, see page 75), Spanish baked fish (*below*, see page 76).

Lentil and split pea loaf   See page 57

Serves 4–6
4 servings
Each serving: 300 Cals/1,240 kJ, 30 g (3 units) carbohydrate, 12 g fibre, 18 g protein, 11 g fat
6 servings
Each serving: 200 Cals/830 kJ, 20 g (2 units) carbohydrate, 8 g fibre, 12 g protein, 7 g fat

100 g/3½ oz split peas
100 g/3½ oz brown lentils
6 tbsp chopped parsley
½ tsp dried mixed herbs
500 ml/18 fl oz stock or vegetable
  water
30 ml/2 tbsp corn oil
1 medium-sized onion, chopped
2 tbsp chopped green peppers
2 medium-sized carrots, diced
2 sticks celery, chopped
1 clove garlic, crushed
1 egg, beaten
30 g/4 tbsp natural bran flakes
60 g/2 oz minced cooked ham
seasoning

Heat the oven to 190°C/375°F/gas 5.
Cook the lentils and peas together with herbs in the stock until soft (see page 36) and all the liquid has been absorbed.
Heat the oil in a large pan and gently cook all the remaining vegetables with the lid on for 20–25 minutes, giving the pan an occasional shake or stir. The vegetables should be lightly browned. Stir into the lentil and bean mixture. Stir in the egg, bran flakes and chopped ham and season well.
Put the mixture into a greased 450-g (1-lb) loaf tin or suitable baking dish, cover with foil or a lid, and bake for 40–45 minutes.

Serving suggestions
If serving hot, Tomato sauce I (see page 117) and any fresh vegetables may accompany it. When serving cold the top may be decorated with sliced radishes and thin slices of peppers, and a crisp green salad served as an accompaniment.

FISH, POULTRY AND MEAT

FISH

Crispie-topped fish pie

Serves 4
Each serving: 360 Cals/1,510 kJ, 40 g (4 units) carbohydrate, 6 g **fibre,** 24 g protein, 12 g fat

340 g/¾ lb filleted white fish
15 g/½ oz polyunsaturated margarine
20 g/2 tbsp wholemeal flour
250 ml/9 fl oz hot skimmed milk
30 ml/2 tbsp tomato ketchup
seasoning

225 g/8 oz corn kernels
180 g/6 oz sliced wholemeal bread
spread with
30 g/1 oz polyunsaturated margarine
30 ml/2 tbsp skimmed milk

Heat the oven to 200°C/400°F/gas 6.
Poach the fish in the milk until tender. Remove the fish and flake it. Melt the margarine over a low heat then stir in the flour. Remove from the heat and gradually stir in the hot milk, bring to the boil, stirring continually, until the sauce thickens. Simmer for 2 minutes, still stirring. Stir in the tomato ketchup, seasoning, corn and fish. Pour into a 1-litre (2-pint) dish. Cut each slice of bread into four triangles and place on top of the fish mixture, margarine side uppermost. Brush with cold skimmed milk and bake for 25–30 minutes until the bread is crisp.

Smoked fish lasagne

Serves 6–8
6 servings
Each serving: 410 Cals/1,740 kJ, 60 g (6 units) carbohydrate, 8 g **fibre,** 31 g protein, 9 g fat
8 servings
Each serving: 310 Cals/1,310 kJ, 40 g (4 units) carbohydrate, 6 g **fibre,** 23 g protein, 7 g fat

300 g/10½ oz wholemeal lasagne
450 g/1 lb smoked haddock
1 bay leaf
sprig parsley
500 ml/18 fl oz skimmed milk
pepper

4 sticks celery, chopped
225 g/8 oz corn kernels
Sauce:
80 g/8 tbsp wholemeal flour
45 g/1½ oz polyunsaturated margarine

Boil the lasagne in salted water until half-cooked. Drain carefully.

Heat the oven to 190°C/375°F/gas 5.

Cook the haddock with the bay leaf, parsley, milk and pepper until the fish starts to flake. Strain the liquid and reserve for the sauce. Discard the herbs and remove any bones and skin from fish and flake.

While the fish and lasagne are cooking, boil the celery until cooked. Drain and reserve 450 ml/¾ pt of the water for the sauce. Mix together flaked fish, celery and corn. Make the sauce (see page 67) using the milk and vegetable water. Place a thin layer of the fish mixture in a non-stick dish then a layer of lasagne, then a layer of sauce. Repeat twice, finally coating with the remainder of the sauce.* Bake for 30–35 minutes.

Kedgeree

Serves 4

Each serving: 300 Cals/1,270 kJ, 30 g (3 units) carbohydrate, 3 g fibre, 19 g protein, 12 g fat

170 g/6 oz brown rice
225 g/8 oz cooked smoked fish, skinned,
  boned and flaked
15 g/½ oz polyunsaturated margarine

seasoning
1 hard-boiled egg, yolk and white of
  egg chopped separately
2 tbsp chopped parsley

Cook the rice (see page 37). Stir in the fish, margarine and seasoning. Mix well and heat through. Spoon on to a serving dish and garnish with egg yolk, white and parsley.

Baked stuffed sole

Serves 4

Each serving: 150 Cals/630 kJ, 10 g (1 unit) carbohydrate, 2 g fibre, 20 g protein, 5 g fat

400 g/14 oz white fish fillets, skinned
30 ml/2 tbsp skimmed milk
15 g/½ oz wholemeal breadcrumbs
15 g/½ oz polyunsaturated margarine
1 tbsp chopped parsley
lemon wedges
Stuffing:
30 g/1 oz wholemeal breadcrumbs

3 large spring onions, chopped including
  green part
30 g/1 oz shrimps, chopped
seasoning
30 ml/2 tbsp skimmed milk

---

* This dish can be prepared in advance to this stage, covered and stored in the refrigerator, but allow 40–45 minutes for final cooking.

Heat the oven to 180°C/350°F/gas 4.
Use a non-stick baking dish or greased baking dish and put in two fish fillets with skinned side up. Mix the dry ingredients for the stuffing and bind with the milk. Spread over the fish, cover with the remaining fillets, brush with the milk and sprinkle the crumbs on top. Dot with margarine and bake in the oven for 20–25 minutes. Garnish with the parsley and lemon wedges.

Tuna Provençal See page 70

Serves 4–6
4 servings
Each serving: 450 Cals/1,880 kJ, 50 g (5 units) carbohydrate, 8 g fibre, 21 g protein, 18 g fat
6 servings
Each serving: 300 Cals/1,250 kJ, 40 g (4 units) carbohydrate, 6 g fibre, 14 g protein, 12 g fat

15 ml/1 tbsp corn oil
3 medium-sized onions, sliced
1 clove garlic, crushed
450 g/1 lb tomatoes, chopped (or use canned)
2 tbsp chopped parsley
small sprig fresh tarragon
1½ tbsp oregano

seasoning
900 g/2 lb potatoes, cut in large dice
200-g/7-oz can tuna fish with own liquid, flaked
30 ml/2 tbsp lemon juice
12 black olives, stoned and halved
30 g/1 oz Parmesan cheese, grated

Heat the oven to 190°C/375°F/gas 5
Heat the oil in an oven-proof casserole, and gently cook the onions and garlic for 5 minutes. Stir in the tomatoes, herbs and seasoning and cook for 1–2 minutes. Remove from the casserole. Place half the potatoes in the casserole and cover with half the tuna, lemon juice and half the tomato mixture. Repeat this layering of potato, tuna and tomato. Cover and cook for 1½ hours until the potatoes are tender. Remove the lid, sprinkle with olives and cheese, and serve.

Fish crumble

Serves 4
Each serving: 300 Cals/1,270 kJ, 20 g (2 units) carbohydrate, 7 g fibre, 15 g protein, 20 g fat

15 ml/1 tbsp corn oil
1 medium-sized onion, chopped
1 clove garlic, crushed
2 medium-sized green peppers, sliced
115 g/4 oz mushrooms, sliced
2 medium-sized tomatoes
seasoning

225 g/8 oz mackerel, flaked
Crumble:
30 g/1 oz polyunsaturated margarine
60 g/6 tbsp wholemeal flour
30 g/4 tbsp natural bran flakes
seasoning

Heat the oven to 180°/350°F/gas 4.

Heat the oil and gently fry the onion and garlic until soft, add the peppers, mushrooms and tomatoes, season well and cook gently for 5 minutes. Remove from the heat. Place half the mixture in a baking dish, cover with the fish and spoon over the remainder of vegetable mixture.

For the crumble, rub the margarine into the dry ingredients, season and cover the vegetable mixture. Bake for 20–30 minutes or until golden brown.

Spanish baked fish   See page 70

Serves 4
Each serving: 140 Cals/590 kJ, 10 g (1 unit) carbohydrate, 2 g fibre, 19 g protein, 2 g fat

5 ml/1 tsp corn oil
1 Spanish onion, chopped
400 g/14 oz canned tomatoes
seasoning
1½ tsp marjoram
1 small canned (or ½ a fresh) red pepper, chopped

125 ml/4 fl oz dry white wine or cider
5 g/2 tsp cornflour
6 green olives, stoned and sliced
1 tbsp capers
1 tbsp chopped parsley
400 g/14 oz white fish fillets

Heat the oil and cook the onion slowly until soft. Add the tomatoes, seasoning, marjoram, pepper and wine. Cover and simmer 20 minutes. Heat the oven to 200°C/400°F/gas 6. Blend the cornflour with 15 ml/1 tbsp cold water, stir into the sauce and simmer for 2 minutes. Add half the olives, capers and parsley. Place the fish in a non-stick greased baking dish and pour the sauce over. Bake for 20–25 minutes or until fish flakes easily, basting with the sauce after 10 minutes and immediately prior to serving. Serve decorated with the remaining olives, capers and parsley.

Fish with shallots and garlic

Serves 4
Each serving: 150 Cals/620 kJ, negligible (0 units) carbohydrate, 1 g fibre 18 g protein, 4 g fat

15 ml/1 tbsp corn oil
2 tsp chopped parsley
2 shallots or small onions, finely chopped (or grated)
400 g/14 oz white fish fillets, skinned

seasoning
1 clove garlic, crushed
2 medium-sized tomatoes, sliced
125 ml/5 fl oz white wine or cider
10 g/3 tbsp wholemeal breadcrumbs

Heat the oven to 180°C/350°F/gas 4.

Heat a baking dish large enough to hold the fillets when placed side-by-side, then grease lightly with some of the oil;

sprinkle the base with the parsley and 1 tsp of shallot or onion and leave for about 5 minutes to let the flavours mix. Place the fish in the dish and sprinkle with salt, pepper, garlic and remaining shallot or onion, then top each piece with thinly sliced tomatoes. Pour over the wine or cider, sprinkle over the remaining oil then the breadcrumbs and bake for 15–20 minutes.

Fish pie

Serves 4–6
4 servings
Each serving: 390 Cals/1,640 kJ, 70 g (7 units) carbohydrate, 19 g fibre, 26 g protein, 3 g fat
6 servings
Each serving: 260 Cals/1,090 kJ, 50 g (5 units) carbohydrate, 12 g fibre, 17 g protein, 2 g fat

200 g/7 oz haricot beans, soaked (see page 36)
200 g/7 oz cooked white fish, flaked
15 ml/1 tbsp lemon juice
2 tbsp chopped parsley
225 g/8 oz mixed vegetables*

275 ml/10 fl oz canned asparagus soup (reconstituted volume if condensed soup used)
4 medium-sized tomatoes, thinly sliced
Topping:
680 g/1½ lb hot mashed potato
90 ml/6 tbsp skimmed milk

Cook the beans (see page 36) then lightly mash with a fork. Mix with the fish, lemon juice, parsley and mixed vegetables. Heat the soup, stir in the vegetable mixture and heat through for 5–10 minutes, then turn into a hot pie dish and cover with the sliced tomatoes. Mash the potato with 60 ml/4 tbsp of the milk and cover the tomatoes. Brush the remaining milk over the potato and brown under a hot grill.

Alternatively, the pie can be prepared in advance, cooled, kept in the refrigerator then cooked in a moderatly hot oven 190°C/375°F/gas 5 for 25–30 minutes.

---

* Calculated as equal amounts of carrot, corn kernels, peas and broad beans.

POULTRY

Chicken lasagne

Serves 4

Each serving: 380 Cals/1,600 kJ, 40 g (4 units) carbohydrate, 9 g **fibre,** 26 g protein, 13 g fat

140 g/5 oz wholemeal lasagne
15 ml/1 tbsp corn oil
1 large onion, chopped
1 clove garlic, crushed
400 g/14 oz tomatoes
1 tbsp marjoram, chopped
4 outer stalks celery, diced and lightly cooked
6 tbsp chopped green pepper
170 g/6 oz cooked chicken, diced
seasoning
30 g/1 oz Parmesan cheese, grated

Country bechamel sauce:
1 small onion, chopped
small piece carrot, chopped
small piece turnip, chopped
½ bay leaf
½ blade of mace
425 ml/¾ pt skimmed milk
30 g/3 tbsp wholemeal flour
15 g/½ oz polyunsaturated margarine
seasoning
Garnish:
paprika

Heat the oven to 190°C/375°F/gas 5.

Cook the lasagne in boiling salted water until half-cooked, drain carefully.

Heat the oil and cook the onion and garlic for 5 minutes until soft. Add the tomatoes, marjoram, celery, peppers, chicken and seasoning and cook for 5 minutes.

To make the sauce, simmer the vegetables, bay leaf and mace in nearly all the milk for 15 minutes. Remove the bay leaf and mace and mix the ingredients in a blender. Return to the pan and bring to the boil.

Meanwhile, blend the flour with the remaining milk. Stir the hot milk into the flour, add the margarine and seasonings, return to pan and cook gently for a few minutes. Place chicken mixture, bechamel sauce and lasagne in alternate layers in a dish, finishing with sauce. Scatter the cheese evenly over the top * and cook for 30–35 minutes. Sprinkle a little paprika on top and serve.

---

* This dish can be prepared in advance to this stage, covered and stored in the refrigerator, but allow 40–45 minutes for the final cooking.

OPPOSITE: Navarin of lamb (*above*, see page 88), Quick pork and peas with brown rice (*below*, see page 90).
OVERLEAF: Chicken Chinese style (see page 84).

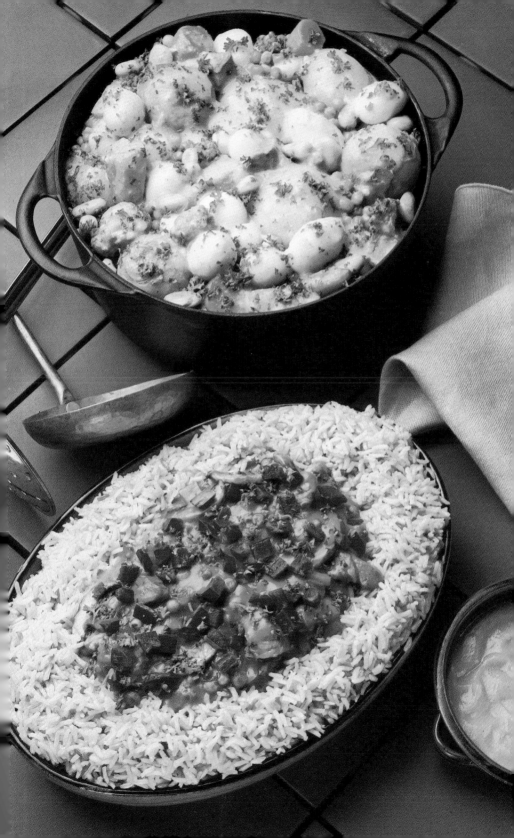

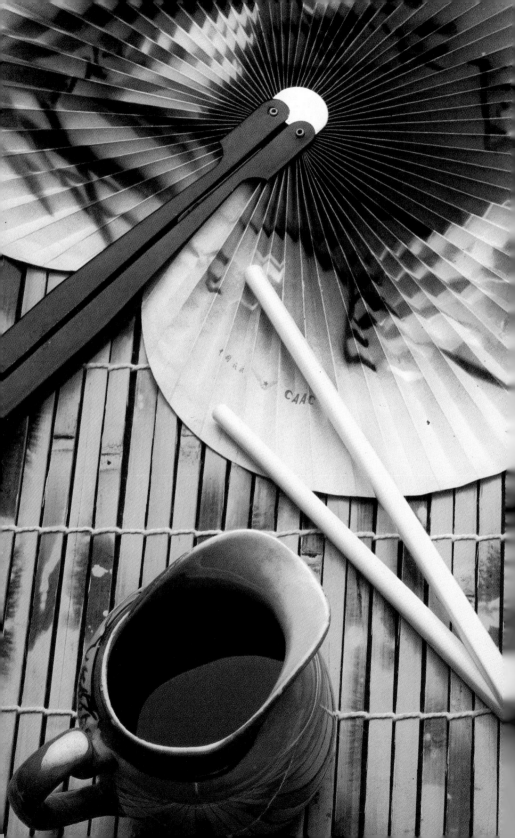

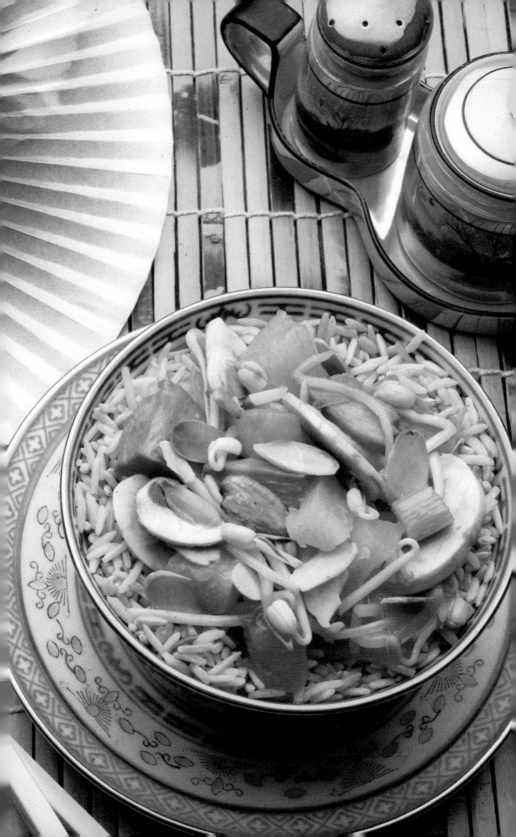

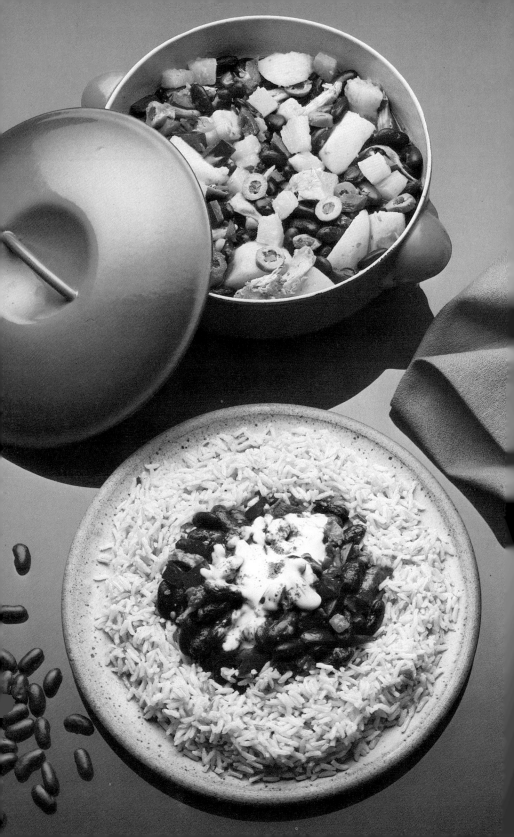

Caribbean chicken See page 82

Serves 4–6
4 servings
Each serving: 640 Cals/2,690 kJ, 90 g (9 units) carbohydrate, 34 g fibre, 50 g protein, 11 g fat
6 servings
Each serving: 430 Cals/1,800 kJ, 60 g (6 units) carbohydrate, 23 g fibre, 33 g protein, 7 g fat

450 g/1 lb red kidney beans, soaked (see page 36)
15 ml/1 tbsp corn oil
340 g/¾ lb chicken, cut in neat cubes
2 medium-sized onions, finely chopped
1 clove garlic, crushed
500 ml/18 fl oz chicken stock
2 medium-sized red peppers, chopped
60 g/2 oz lean cooked ham, chopped
4 medium-sized tomatoes, chopped (or use canned)
30 g/1 oz seedless raisins, roughly chopped
2 tbsp capers, roughly chopped
1½ tbsp oregano
¼ tsp (approx) Tabasco sauce
30 ml/2 tbsp tomato purée
600 g/1 lb 5 oz potatoes, quartered
seasoning
100 g/3½ oz fresh pineapple or pineapple canned without added sugar, chopped
10 stuffed olives, sliced

Cook the beans (see page 36).
Meanwhile, heat the oil and gently cook the chicken until lightly browned. Remove with a slotted spoon and add the onions, garlic and 60 ml/4 tbsp stock. Stir well, lower the heat and cook slowly for 15–20 minutes until the onion is tender but not brown. Mix in the peppers, ham, tomatoes, raisins, capers, oregano, Tabasco, tomato purée, seasonings, remaining stock and the chicken, bring to the boil then simmer for 20 minutes. Add the potatoes and cooked beans, return to the boil, lower the heat and simmer for 20–30 minutes until the potatoes are cooked. Sprinkle the pineapple over the top and press partly down into the mixture, then sprinkle over the olives and serve.

Chicken and rice casserole

Serves 4–6
4 servings
Each serving: 400 Cals/1,680 kJ, 70 g (7 units) carbohydrate, 9 g fibre, 24 g protein, 5 g fat
6 servings
Each serving: 270 Cals/1,120 kJ, 40 g (4 units) carbohydrate, 6 g fibre, 16 g protein, 4 g fat ➡

Caribbean chicken (*above*), Beef and bean goulash (*below*, see page 86).

300 g/10½ oz long-grain brown rice
300 g/10½ oz uncooked chicken, chopped
2 medium-sized onions, chopped
340 g/12 oz mixed vegetables (see Quick chicken charlotte below)
1 tsp curry powder
10–15 ml/2–3 tsp soy sauce
seasoning
1 litre/1¾ pts boiling chicken stock
2 tbsp chopped parsley

Heat the oven to 180°C/350°F/gas 4.

Mix the rice, meat and vegetables together in casserole. Mix the curry powder, soy sauce and seasoning with the stock and stir into rice mixture. Cover and cook for 1¼–1½ hours until the rice has absorbed the stock and is tender. Stir in half the parsley, sprinkle the remainder on top and serve.

Quick chicken charlotte

Serves 4
Each serving: 370 Cals/1,570 kJ, 40 g (4 units) carbohydrate, 7 g fibre, 30 g protein, 12 g fat

100 g/3½ oz wholemeal breadcrumbs mixed with
100 g/3½ oz rolled oats
340 g/12 oz cooked chicken, neatly diced
mixed vegetables, chopped eg:
  60 g/2 oz celery
  60 g/2 oz carrots
  60 g/2 oz turnip
60 g/2 oz peas
60 g/2 oz broad beans
60 g/2 oz corn kernels
1 tbsp mixed herbs
seasoning
300 g/10½ oz canned mushroom soup (reconstituted volume if condensed soup used)
150 ml/5 fl oz water

Heat the oven to 200°C/400°F/gas 6.

Grease a baking dish and sprinkle the base with one-third of the mixed breadcrumbs and oats. Mix together the chicken, vegetables and herbs and season. Arrange on the crumb-and-oat mixture and pour in the soup and water. Cover with the remaining crumb-and-oat mixture and bake for 45 minutes.

Chicken Chinese style See pages 80–1

Serves 4
Each serving: 220 Cals/940 kJ, 20 g (2 units) carbohydrate, 8 g fibre, 17 g protein, 9 g fat

225 g/½ lb chicken
15 ml/1 tbsp corn oil
seasoning
30 ml/2 tbsp soy sauce
100 g/3½ oz fresh pineapple canned without added sugar, chopped
510 g/16 oz beansprouts
4 sticks celery, sliced
115 g/4 oz mushrooms, sliced
250 ml/9 fl oz chicken stock
10 g/1 tbsp wholemeal flour
15 g/½ oz flaked almonds, toasted
225 g/8 oz cooked long-grain brown rice (75 g/2½ oz dry weight)

Cut the chicken in neat 15-mm (½-in) pieces. Heat the oil, add the chicken and seasoning and cook gently for 15 minutes. Stir in the soy sauce, pineapple, beansprouts, celery, mushrooms and stock. Cover tightly, bring to the boil and simmer for 5 minutes. Blend the flour with a little water and stir into the chicken. Bring to simmering point stirring constantly, then simmer for 5 minutes. Adjust seasoning if necessary, sprinkle on the toasted almonds and serve with the rice.

MEAT

Beef à la Créole

Serves 6
Each serving: 300 Cals/1,250 kJ, 40 g (4 units) carbohydrate, 8 g fibre, 14 g protein, 4 g fat

15 ml/1 tbsp corn oil	*1 tbsp each oregano and basil*
2 large onions, sliced	*good pinch cayenne*
225 g/½ lb lean stewing steak, diced	*seasoning*
3 medium-sized carrots, cubed	*125 ml/4 fl oz red wine*
3 large outer sticks celery, sliced	*225 g/½ lb okra, sliced*
15 ml/1 tbsp tomato purée	*400 g/14 oz cooked long-grain brown*
a few sprigs thyme and parsley	*rice (140 g/5 oz dry weight)*

Heat the oil and cook the onions gently for 5 minutes. Add a few tbsp stock, mix well and stir for about 5 minutes. Stir in the beef and stir well to coat with the onions. Stir in the celery, carrots, tomato purée, herbs, seasoning and wine and simmer gently for about 1¾ hours. Add the okra and cook for about ½ hour. If there is too much juice, turn up the heat, remove the lid and let some of the liquid evaporate. If it should be too concentrated, add a little meat stock or water and heat through. Serve with the brown rice.

Country casserole

Serves 4
Each serving: 240 Cals/990 kJ, 20 g (2 units) carbohydrate, 5 g fibre, 21 g protein, 8 g fat

10 ml/2 tsp corn oil	*1 tbsp oregano*
2 large onions, chopped	*seasoning*
1 clove garlic, crushed	*2 medium-sized red peppers*
340 g/¾ lb lean stewing beef, diced	*225 g/8 oz corn kernels*
375 ml/13 fl oz beef stock	*4 tbsp chopped parsley*

Heat the oven to 170°C/325°F/gas 3.
   Heat the oil and gently cook the onion and garlic for 10

minutes. Add the beef and cook for 5 minutes, stirring well. Stir in the stock, oregano and seasoning. Cover and cook for 2–2¼ hours until the meat is tender. Stir in the peppers and corn and cook for ¼ hour. Garnish liberally with chopped parsley and serve.

This dish may also be cooked on a very low heat on top of the stove.

Meatballs in curry sauce with brown rice and bananas

Serves 4
Each serving: 590 Cals/2,490 kJ, 100 g (10 units) carbohydrate, 33 g fibre, 35 g protein, 10 g fat

300 g/10½ oz haricot beans, soaked (see page 36)
200 g/7 oz lean meat, minced
1 medium-sized onion, finely chopped
1 clove garlic, crushed
30 g/1 oz wholemeal bread, crumbed
seasoning
small pinch ground cinnamon, ground cloves and ground cardamoms

1 small egg, beaten with 15 ml/1 tbsp cold water
60 g/8 tbsp coarse, natural bran flakes
Curry sauce (see page 116, using 250 ml/9 fl oz stock)
450 g/1 lb cooked long-grain brown rice (140 g/5 oz dry weight)
400 g/14 oz bananas

Cook the beans (see page 36). Drain and dry thoroughly then mash well with a fork and mix with the meat, onion, garlic, breadcrumbs, seasoning and spices. Knead well and divide into 12 small balls. Roll in the bran flakes, then dip in the beaten egg and finally in the bran flakes, pressing the coating well into the balls. Grill until browned, add to the Curry sauce and simmer gently for 10 minutes giving the saucepan an occasional shake, but do not stir as this may break up the meatballs. Pile the rice on a hot serving dish, making a well in the centre for the curry mixture. Serve the bananas separately.

Beef and bean goulash   See page 82

Serves 4–6
4 servings
Each serving: 330 Cals/1,370 kJ, 40 g (4 units) carbohydrate, 16 g fibre, 27 g protein, 8 g fat
6 servings
Each serving: 220 Cals/910 kJ, 30 g (3 units) carbohydrate, 11 g fibre, 18 g protein, 5 g fat

15 ml/1 tbsp corn oil
2 large onions, chopped
500 ml/18 fl oz meat stock
1 clove garlic, crushed
4 tsp paprika pepper
200 g/7 oz lean stewing steak*, cut in
   neat pieces
30 g/3 tbsp wholemeal flour

400 g/14 oz canned tomatoes
1 tbsp marjoram
200 g/7 oz red kidney beans, soaked
   (see page 36)
3 medium-sized red peppers
seasoning
150 ml/5 fl oz low-fat plain yoghurt

Heat the oil and stir in the onions, add a few tbsp stock and stir for about 5 minutes, until the onions begin to soften and brown slightly. Stir in the garlic and paprika then stir in the meat. Sprinkle·on the flour, then stir in the tomatoes, marjoram and remaining stock and simmer for 1 hour. Add the beans and cook for about 45 minutes. Add the peppers and salt and cook for about 15 minutes until the meat and beans are tender. Serve with the yoghurt spooned over.

Shepherd's pie

Serves 4
Each serving: 440 Cals/1,840 kJ, 70 g (7 units) carbohydrate, 18 g fibre, 33 g protein, 6 g fat

200 g/7 oz haricot beans, soaked (see
   page 36)
300 g/10½ oz canned tomato soup
   (reconstituted volume if condensed)
1 Spanish onion, finely chopped
1 medium-sized red pepper, finely
   chopped
60-g/2-oz slice wholemeal bread,
   crumbled

200 g/7 oz cooked lean meat, minced
4 tbsp chopped parsley
seasoning
450 g/1 lb potatoes
60 g/2 oz red lentils
pinch nutmeg
30 ml/2 tbsp skimmed milk

Cook the beans (see page 36). Mix the soup, onion and pepper in a pan and simmer gently for 10 minutes. Add the bread and work with a cooking spoon until the ingredients are well mixed. Stir in the meat and beans, bring up to the boil and heat through thoroughly, stirring occasionally. Mix in the parsley and seasoning. Transfer to a pie dish.

Meanwhile, cook the potatoes and lentils together then mash with the nutmeg and cover the pie. Brush with the milk,† brown lightly under the grill and serve.

---

* Veal or lamb can be used instead of beef.

† The pie can be made to this stage, left to cool, covered and refrigerated. Bake in a moderately hot oven for 25–30 minutes when required.

Navarin of lamb   See page 79

Serves 4–6
4 servings
Each serving: 370 Cals/1,540 kJ, 40 g (4 units) carbohydrate, 14 g
fibre, 27 g protein, 12 g fat
6 servings
Each serving: 240 Cals/1,030 kJ, 30 g (3 units) carbohydrate, 9 g
fibre, 18 g protein, 8 g fat

340 g/¾ lb lean stewing lamb	*8 small carrots*
15 ml/1 tbsp corn oil	*600 g/1 lb 5 oz potatoes*
20 g/2 tbsp wholemeal flour	*8 small white turnips*
1 clove garlic, crushed	*1 tbsp rosemary*
seasoning	*225 g/8 oz peas*
500 ml/18 fl oz water	*225 g/8 oz broad beans*
12 button onions	*4 tbsp chopped parsley*

Trim the excess fat from the meat. Cut the meat into small
neat pieces. Heat the oil and fry the meat until golden brown.
Sprinkle the flour, garlic and seasoning over the meat and
cook, stirring, until the meat and flour are well browned.
Slowly pour in the water and stir until it boils. Cover and
simmer for 1 hour. Remove from the heat, leave to cool and
skim off the surface fat. Return to the heat. Add the onions,
carrots, turnips, potatoes and rosemary and simmer for 30
minutes. Add the peas and beans and cook for 10–15 minutes,
until the ingredients are tender. Stir in the parsley and serve.

Haricot lamb

Serves 4
Each serving: 310 Cals/1,300 kJ, 40 g (4 units) carbohydrate, 17 g
fibre, 25 g protein, 8 g fat

225 g/½ lb lean stewing lamb	*seasoning*
10 ml/2 tsp oil	*2 medium-sized carrots, chopped*
2 medium-sized onions, sliced	*200 g/7 oz swede or turnip, chopped*
200 g/7 oz haricot beans, soaked (see	*30 g/3 tbsp wholemeal flour*
page 36)	*2 tbsp chopped parsley*
375 ml/13 fl oz water	

Trim excess fat from the meat. Cut the meat into small, neat
pieces. Heat the oil and fry the onion until golden brown.
Draw the onion to the side of the pan and fry the meat until
lightly browned. Add the beans, water and seasoning and boil
for 10 minutes, then simmer for 1–1¼ hours. Add the carrots
and swede or turnip and cook for ½–¾ hour until very tender.
Blend the flour with 30 ml/2 tbsp cold water, add a little hot
gravy from the casserole and stir into the stew. Cook for 5
minutes, garnish with the parsley and serve.

This casserole can also be cooked in a slow oven for approximately 2 hours.

Irish stew

Serves 4
Each serving: 340 Cals/1,410 kJ, 50 g (5 units) carbohydrate, 11 g fibre, 21 g protein, 5 g fat

225 g/½ lb lean stewing lamb
2 large Spanish onions
seasoning
375 ml/15 fl oz water
750 g/1¾ lb potatoes, cut in half

2 medium-sized carrots, chopped
3 outer stalks celery, chopped
225 g/8 oz peas
2 tbsp chopped parsley

Trim the excess fat off the meat. Cut the meat into small neat pieces, and put in large pan with the onion and seasoning. Add the water, cover with close-fitting lid and cook gently for 1¼ hours, shaking occasionally. Add the potatoes, carrots and celery and cook for ¾ hour. Add the peas and cook for 10 minutes, sprinkle the parsley on top and serve.

The casserole can also be cooked in a slow oven for approximately 2 hours.

Bean and lamb stew

Serves 4–6
4 servings
Each serving: 310 Cals/1,300 kJ, 30 g (3 units) carbohydrate, 16 g fibre, 25 g protein, 9 g fat
6 servings
Each serving: 210 Cals/860 kJ, 20 g (2 units) carbohydrate, 11 g fibre, 17 g protein, 6 g fat

225 g/8 oz red kidney beans, soaked
  (see page 36)
15 ml/1 tbsp corn oil
1 large onion, chopped
200 g/7 oz lean lamb, diced
10 g/1 tbsp wholemeal flour
500 ml/18 fl oz water

60 ml/4 tbsp tomato purée
½ tsp powdered cumin
1 small bay leaf
sprig rosemary or ½ tsp dried rosemary
4 medium-sized tomatoes, halved
seasoning
2 tbsp finely chopped spring onions

Heat the oil and fry the onion until transparent. Toss the lamb in flour and add to the casserole. Cook for 10 minutes, stirring occasionally. Add the beans and water, stir in the tomato purée, cumin, bay leaf and rosemary. Cover, boil for 10 minutes, then simmer for 1 hour. Place the tomatoes (cut side up) on top, season, replace the lid and cook gently for 20 minutes. Sprinkle the spring onions over the top and serve.

Quick pork and peas with brown rice

See page 79

Serves 4
Each serving: 530 Cals/2,240 kJ, 90 g (9 units) carbohydrate, 13 g fibre, 25 g protein, 10 g fat

300 g/10½ oz long-grain brown rice
40 g/4 tbsp wholemeal flour
seasoning
200 g/7 oz lean pork, chopped
15 ml/1 tbsp corn oil
1 chicken stock cube
1½ tbsp sage
375 ml/13 fl oz cider or dry white wine

30 ml/2 tbsp tomato purée
115 g/4 oz mushrooms, sliced
400 g/14 oz peas
125 ml/4 fl oz Apple sauce (see page 116)
2 tbsp chopped parsley
1 small red pepper, chopped

Cook the rice (see page 37). Season the flour and coat the meat. Heat the oil and cook the onions and meat for 5 minutes, stirring. Stir in any remaining flour, the stock cube, sage, cider or wine and tomato purée. Bring to the boil then simmer for 20 minutes. Add the mushrooms and peas and cook for 10 minutes. Adjust seasoning if necessary. Arrange the rice around the outside of a serving dish. Spoon the pork into the centre and sprinkle on the peppers and parsley. Serve the Apple sauce separately.

BAKING

In yeast cookery ensure that all utensils used are warm and the area for preparation is free from cold draughts.

Wholemeal soda bread

Makes 2 loaves
Each 30 g/1 oz slice: 60 Cals/250 kJ, 10 g (1 unit) carbohydrate, 2 g fibre, 3 g protein, negligible fat

450 g/1 lb wholemeal flour
1 tsp salt
1 tsp cream of tartar

1 tsp bicarbonate of soda
250 ml/9 fl oz buttermilk

Heat the oven to 220°C/425°F/gas 7.
    Mix all the dry ingredients together. Add the buttermilk and

---

Quick wholemeal bread (*above*, see page 93), Quick wholemeal rolls (*below left*, see page 93), Bran muffins (*below right*, see page 94).

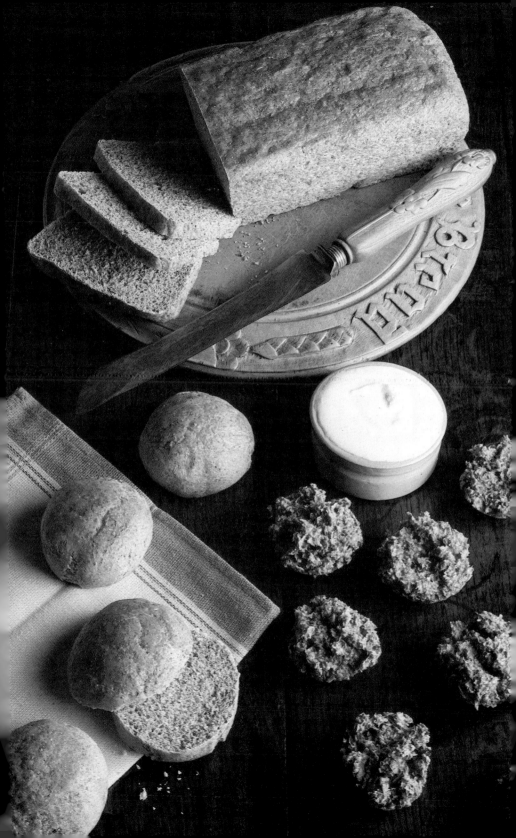

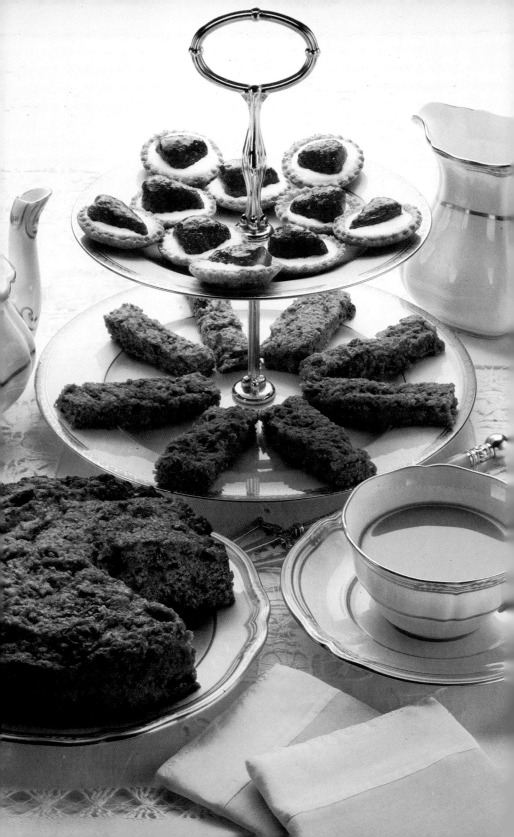

mix to a light elastic dough. Divide the mixture in two and shape into rounds. Place on a greased baking tray and mark into four sections with a knife. Bake for 30–40 minutes until firm and well browned. Cool on a wire rack. For a softer crust wrap in a tea-towel to cool.

This recipe can also be made using 250 ml/10 fl oz skimmed milk instead of buttermilk and using 2 tsp cream of tartar.

Quick wholemeal bread See page 91

Makes 1 loaf
Each 30 g/1 oz slice: 55 Cals/230 kJ, 10 g (1 unit) carbohydrate, 2 g fibre, 2 g protein, 1 g fat

1 tsp sugar
1½ tsp dried yeast or
15 g/½ oz fresh yeast
450 g/1 lb wholemeal flour

1 tsp salt
15 g/1 tbsp polyunsaturated margarine
250 ml/9 fl oz (approx) lukewarm water

Dissolve the sugar in lukewarm water, stir into the yeast and leave in a warm place for 10–15 minutes until frothy. In a large bowl, mix the flour with the salt and rub in the margarine. Beat the yeast liquid into the flour to form a dough. Turn onto a lightly floured surface and knead by folding the dough towards you, then pushing away with the palm of the hand for about 10 minutes, until firm and elastic. Place the dough in bowl, cover with lightly oiled polythene and leave to rise until double in size (1–1½ hours in a warm place). Turn the dough onto a lightly floured surface and knead for about 2 minutes until firm. Shape to fit a lightly greased 450-g/1-lb loaf tin, cover with oiled polythene and leave in a warm place for about 45 minutes until the dough is just rounded over the top of the tin.

Heat the oven to 230°C/450°F/gas 8. Bake the loaf for 30–40 minutes until golden brown and sounds hollow if tapped underneath. Cool on a wire tray.

Variations
Rolls (see page 91) Divide the 450 g/1 lb wholemeal bread recipe dough in 12 and press into small rolls. Place on a floured baking tray 1.5 cm (¾ in) apart for soft-sided rolls or 2.5 cm (1 in) apart for crusty rolls. Cover with lightly oiled polythene and leave in a warm place until doubled in size. Bake at 230°C/450°F/gas 8 for 20–25 minutes.

French onion bread To the 450 g/1 lb quantity wholemeal yeast bread recipe, add 3 tbsp finely chopped onion plus 1

Strawberry tartlets (*top*, see page 101), Wholesome fingers (*centre*, see page 97), Rhubarb and date cake (*bottom*, see page 98).

crushed garlic clove sautéed in 15 ml/1 tbsp corn oil, to the yeast, sugar and water mixture when it has become frothy.

Instead of baking the loaf in a tin, shape into an oval or baton shape and place on a non-stick baking sheet. Make small diagonal cuts on top before covering and leaving to rise. Brush the surface with equal quantities of beaten egg white and water. Bake on the middle shelf of the oven at 190°/375°F/gas 5 for 25–30 minutes. Cool on a wire tray.

Breadsticks   These can be made by reserving part of the mixed yeast dough at the stage where the dough has risen to double its size.

Knead the dough on a floured board and roll out to 20 × 22.5 cm (8 × 9 in). Cut into strips about 1 cm (½ in) wide and roll each into a stick. Place on a lightly greased tray and bake in a hot oven until crisp.

Fruity yeast bread

Makes 2 small loaves
Each 30 g/1 oz slice: 60 Cals/250 kJ, 10 g (1 unit) carbohydrate, 2 g fibre, 2 g protein, 1 g fat

150 ml/5 fl oz skimmed milk	*2 tsp salt*
150 ml/5 fl oz hot water	*30 g/1 oz polyunsaturated margarine*
1 tsp sugar	*60 g/2 oz raisins*
1½ tsp dried yeast or ½ oz fresh yeast	*60 g/2 oz currants*
450 g/1 lb wholemeal flour	

Mix the milk and water. Add the sugar and yeast and leave for 5–10 minutes until frothy. Mix the flour and salt and rub in margarine. Add yeast mixture and mix to a dough. Knead well on a lightly floured surface for 10 minutes. Work in the fruit. Divide into two and shape to fill two greased 450-g (1-lb) loaf tins. Cover with greased polythene and leave in a warm place for about 30–35 minutes or 12 hours in the refrigerator.

Heat the oven to 230°C/450°F/gas 8. Bake the loaves for about 45 minutes or until well browned and sound hollow when tapped underneath. Cool on a wire rack.

Bran muffins   See page 91

Makes 24
Each muffin: 70 Cals/290 kJ, 10 g (1 unit) carbohydrate, 3 g fibre, 3 g protein, 2 g fat

250 g/9 oz wholemeal flour	*2 medium-sized eggs*
115 g/4 oz natural bran flakes	*425 ml/¾ pt skimmed milk*
25 g/5 tsp baking powder	*15 ml/1 tbsp corn oil*
½ tsp mixed spice	*115 g/4 oz dates, chopped*
1 tsp salt	

Heat the oven to 200°C/400°F/gas 6.

Mix the flour, bran flakes, baking powder, mixed spice and salt together. Beat the eggs, milk and oil together and add with the dates to the dry ingredients, stirring only sufficiently to mix evenly. Fill 24 non-stick patty tins and bake for 15–20 minutes or until brown. Serve with low-fat cheese.

Sweet spiced bran muffins

Makes 15
Each muffin: 60 Cals/270 kJ, 10 g (1 unit) carbohydrate, 3 g fibre, 3 g protein, 1 g fat

30 g/1 oz skimmed-milk powder
15 g/3 tsp baking powder
1 tsp salt
2 tsp mixed spice
70 g/2½ oz natural bran flakes
155 g/5½ oz wholemeal flour
2 tsp grated orange rind

2 medium-sized eggs, beaten
sugar-free liquid sweetener equivalent
* to 60 g/2 oz sugar*
5 ml/1 tsp corn oil
250 ml/9 fl oz skimmed milk
70 g/2½ oz apple, grated
1 small carrot, finely grated

Heat the oven to 200°C/400°F/gas 6.

Stir together the milk powder, baking powder, salt, spice, bran flakes, flour and orange rind. Mix together the egg, sweetening, oil and milk. Add to the dry ingredients, stirring just sufficiently to blend evenly. Fold in the apple and carrot. Fill paper baking cups or non-stick patty tins two-thirds full and bake for 15–20 minutes until firm and brown.

Savoury bran muffins

Makes 15
Each muffin: 80 Cals/320 kJ, 10 g (1 unit) carbohydrate, 4 g fibre, 5 g protein, 2 g fat

30 g/1 oz skimmed-milk powder
15 g/3 tsp baking powder
1 tsp garlic salt
115 g/4 oz wholemeal flour
60 g/2 oz natural bran flakes
2 medium-sized eggs, beaten
5 ml/1 tsp corn oil

170 g/6 oz haricot beans, cooked and
* puréed*
150 ml/5 fl oz low-fat plain yoghurt
1 tbsp grated onion
125 ml/5 fl oz skimmed milk
½ tsp grated nutmeg

Heat the oven to 200°C/400°F/gas 6.

Stir together the milk powder, baking powder, salt, flour and bran flakes. Mix together the egg, oil, puréed beans, yoghurt, onion, milk and nutmeg. Stir into the dry ingredients and mix until just evenly blended. Fill paper baking cups or non-stick patty tins two-thirds full and bake for 15–20 minutes until firm and brown. Serve hot with one of the savoury spreads (see page 107) or skimmed-milk cheese.   →

Any left over can be stored in a tin, toasted next day and served on their own or with skimmed-milk cheese and garnished with cress.

Wholemeal yoghurt scones

Makes 12

Each scone: 80 Cals/330 kJ, 10 g (1 unit) carbohydrate, 2 g fibre, 3 g protein, 2 g fat

200 g/7 oz wholemeal flour
1 tsp salt
1 tsp bicarbonate of soda
30 g/1 oz polyunsaturated margarine

150 ml/5 fl oz low-fat plain yoghurt
1–2 tsp grated orange or lemon rind
(optional)

Heat the oven to 220°C/425°F/gas 7.

Place the flour, salt and bicarbonate of soda in bowl. Rub in the margarine, then stir in the fruit and rind, if used, and yoghurt to make a soft dough. Roll to 1 cm (½ in) thick and cut into rounds using a 5-cm (2-in) cutter. Place on a baking tray, brush with a little milk and bake for 8–10 minutes.

Wholemeal yoghurt scones with sultanas
Add 30 g/1 oz chopped sultanas or raisins to the rubbed-in mixture.

Wholemeal scones with dates
Add 60g/2 oz chopped dates to the rubbed-in mixture.

Potato scones

Makes 6

Each scone: 60 Cals/250 kJ, 10 g (1 unit) carbohydrate, 1 g fibre, 1 g protein, 1 g fat

200 g/7 oz potatoes (preferably floury),
peeled and sliced
10 g/2 tsp polyunsaturated margarine

1 tsp salt
40 g/4 tbsp wholemeal flour or oatmeal

Cook the potatoes, drain and mash with the margarine and salt. Work in the flour or oatmeal to form a pliable dough. Roll into a very thin round, cut into 6 pieces and place on a hot griddle, electric hot plate or strong frying pan. Cook for 3–4 minutes on each side. Cool in a towel.

Alternatively place on baking tray and cook in a hot oven 220°C/425°F/gas 7 for 5–8 minutes.

Sweet and spicy wholemeal biscuits

Makes 30

Each biscuit: 40 Cals/180 kJ, 5 g (½ unit) carbohydrate, 1 g fibre, 1 g protein, 2 g fat

100 g/3½ oz rolled oats
100 g/3½ oz wholemeal flour
3 tsp mixed spice (optional)
½ tsp salt

70 g/2½ oz polyunsaturated margarine
100 g/3½ oz cold mashed potato
sugar-free liquid sweetener equivalent
to 18 tsp sugar

Heat the oven to 180°C/350°F/gas 4. Grease 2 baking trays.
Mix together the oats, flour, spice (if used) and salt and rub in the margarine. Beat the potato and sweetener together. Mix into the rubbed-in mixture and knead thoroughly until a very stiff dough is formed. Roll out very thinly on a floured board and cut into 30 rounds using a 6-cm (2½-in) plain cutter. Place on the trays and bake for 25–30 minutes until crisp and slightly coloured. Cool on a rack and store in an airtight tin.

Caraway biscuits
Add 4 tsp caraway seed and ½ tsp freshly grated nutmeg.

Orange biscuits
Add finely grated rind of 1 orange (or rind of half an orange and half a lemon) and 2 tsp crushed coriander seeds.

Savoury biscuits
Omit sweetener and mixed spice. Add 1 tbsp grated onion, ½ tsp garlic salt, ¼ tsp dry mustard and pinch cayenne pepper.

Wholesome fingers See page 92

Makes 24
Each finger: 90 Cals/380 kJ, 10 g (1 unit) carbohydrate, 2 g fibre, 2 g protein, 4 g fat

200 g/7 oz wholemeal flour
2 tsp baking powder
pinch salt
100 g/3½ oz polyunsaturated
  margarine
sugar-free liquid sweetener equivalent
  to 60 g/2 oz sugar
70 g/2½ oz mashed potato (or instant,
  reconstituted)

200 g/7 oz grated carrot
100 g/3½ oz cooked and skinned
  chestnuts, finely chopped *
70 g/2½ oz stoneless dates, chopped
70 g/2½ oz sultanas, chopped
¼ tsp ground cinnamon
¼ tsp ground mace
2 medium-sized eggs, beaten

Heat the oven to 180°C/350°F/gas 4.
Mix the flour, baking powder and salt and rub in the margarine. Beat the sweetener into the potatoes and mix into the flour together with the chestnuts, dates, sultanas, carrot and spices. Beat in the eggs to form a fairly stiff consistency. Spread in a non-stick 18 × 27 cm (7 × 11 in) tin and bake for 30–35 minutes. Leave to cool in the tin, then cut into 24 fingers.

---

* Canned sugar-free chestnuts or dried reconstituted chestnuts can be used instead.

Hazelnut crunchies

Makes 20
Each biscuit: 100 Cals/430 kJ, 10 g (1 unit) carbohydrate, 2 g fibre,
3 g protein, 5 g fat

225 g/8 oz wholemeal flour
30 g/1 oz barley flakes
100 g/3½ oz grated hazelnuts
15 g/3 tsp baking powder
pinch salt
75 g/5 tbsp margarine
100 g/3½ oz cold mashed potato

sugar-free liquid sweetener equivalent
to 15 tsp sugar
10 g/2 tsp mixed spice
60 g/2 oz sultanas, chopped
grated rind 1 orange
1 small egg, beaten
30 g/2 tbsp low-fat plain yoghurt

Heat the oven to 200°C/400°F/gas 6. Grease 2 baking trays.
Mix the flour, barley flakes, hazelnuts, baking powder and salt, then rub in the margarine. Beat the potato and sweetener together. Mix into the rubbed-in mixture with the spice, sultanas and orange rind. Add the egg and yoghurt, mixing well to form a stiff consistency. Put the mixture in small rough heaps on the baking tray and bake for 10–15 minutes. Cool on a wire tray and cut into 20 slices.

Rhubarb and date cake   See page 92

Makes 12 slices
Each slice: 140 Cals/590 kJ, 20 g (2 units) carbohydrate, 4 g fibre,
4 g protein, 5 g fat

225 g/8 oz wholemeal flour
15 g/3 tsp baking powder
225 g/8 oz rhubarb, chopped
170 g/6 oz stoneless dates,

chopped
60 g/2 oz polyunsaturated margarine
1 egg, beaten
60 ml/4 tbsp skimmed milk

Heat the oven to 190°C/375°F/gas 5.
Cook the rhubarb for 5–10 minutes. Rub the margarine into the flour and baking powder and stir in the dates and rhubarb. Add the egg and milk and mix well. Put into a cake tin and bake for 1 hour. Divide into 12 slices.

Fruit and nut loaf

Makes 12 slices
Each slice: 120 Cals/510 kJ, 20 g (2 units) carbohydrate, 2 g fibre,
3 g protein, 7 g fat

140 g/5 oz wholemeal flour
pinch salt
½ tsp mixed spice
1 tsp cinnamon
60 g/2 oz polyunsaturated margarine
100 g/3½ oz dessert apple, grated

2 tsp grated orange rind
1 egg, beaten
90 ml/3 fl oz skimmed milk
85 g/3 oz stoneless dates, chopped
45 g/1½ oz pecan nuts or walnuts,
chopped

Heat the oven to 160°C/325°F/gas 3.

Mix the flour, salt and spices. Cream the margarine with a little of the flour mixture and apple and orange rind together. Add the egg and milk to the flour mixture a little at a time and beat well. Fold in the dates and nuts. Bake for 20 minutes and then reduce the temperature to 150°C/300°F/gas 2 for a further 45–60 minutes. Turn onto a wire rack to cool.

DESSERTS

Turkish apricot and orange dessert

Serves 4–6

4 servings

Each serving: 140 Cals/610 kJ, 30 g (3 units) carbohydrate, 15 g fibre, 6 g protein, 1 g fat

6 servings

Each serving: 100 Cals/410 kJ, 20 g (2 units) carbohydrate, 10 g fibre, 4 g protein, 1 g fat

250 g/8¾ oz dried apricots, soaked overnight in
500 ml/18 fl oz water
grated rind 1 orange
remainder of juice from orange (see 'topping')
sugar-free liquid sweetener to taste

Topping:
60 g/2 oz skimmed-milk cheese (see page 32)
85 ml/3 fl oz low-fat plain yoghurt
25 ml/5 tsp orange juice
sugar-free liquid sweetener to taste

Cook the apricots gently in the soaking liquor until tender (about 20–30 minutes). Add the orange rind and juice, allow to cool slightly and sweeten to taste. Reserve 4 or 6 apricots, purée the remainder and pour into individual glasses.

For the topping, purée the cheese, yoghurt, orange juice and sweetener in a blender. Spoon over the apricot purée, place the reserved apricots, rounded-side up, on the centre of each dish. Chill slightly before serving.

Diabetic jelly

Serves 4

Each serving: 10 Cals/40 kJ, negligible (0 units) carbohydrate, negligible fibre, 3 g protein, negligible fat

15 g/3 tsp unflavoured gelatine
425 ml/¾ pt water

150 ml/¼ pt diabetic squash (orange, lemon, lime or low-calorie ginger ale)

Dissolve the gelatine in a little hot (but not boiling) water in a cup. Add the remaining water and squash, pour into a mould or individual moulds or glass dishes and leave to set.

Pears in lime jelly

Serves 4

Each serving: 60 Cals/240 kJ, 10 g (1 unit) carbohydrate, 4 g fibre, 3 g protein, 0 g fat

Make as for plain jelly above using 600 ml/1 pt low-calorie lime squash and 20 g/4 tsp gelatine. When the liquid is cold, add 500 g/ 1 lb 2 oz canned pears without added sugar, drained and chopped. The liquid from the can can be substituted for some of the water.

Spiced summer fruit sundae

Serves 4

Each serving: 80 Cals/340 kJ, 10 g (1 unit) carbohydrate, 9 g fibre, 5 g protein, 1 g fat

115 g/4 oz orange
stick cinnamon (about 5 cm or 2 in)
250 ml/9 fl oz cold water
20 g/2 tbsp wholemeal flour

sugar-free liquid sweetener to taste
450 g/1 lb mixed berry fruits
100 g/3½ oz skimmed-milk cheese
(see page 35)

Coarsely grate or cut matchsticks of orange rind and squeeze the juice. Place the cinnamon stick in a pan with the water and bring to the boil. Blend the flour with a little cold water and gradually stir in the boiled water. Return to the pan and cook for 3–5 minutes until clear. Remove the cinnamon stick, add the fruit and simmer for 2–3 minutes until slightly softened. Remove from the heat and gently mix in the orange juice and sweetener. Cover and chill. Divide between 4 dishes, spoon the cheese on top and garnish with a few shreds of orange rind.

Apple and cherry crunchie

Serves 4

Each serving: 120 Cals/500 kJ, 10 g (1 unit) carbohydrate, 1 g fibre, 10 g protein, 3 g fat

250 g/8 oz skimmed-milk cheese (see page 35)
150 ml/5 fl oz low-fat black-cherry yoghurt

200 g/7 oz red apples, cored and diced
few sprigs mint

Stir cheese into the yoghurt and add the apples. Cover and chill slightly. Serve garnished with sprigs of mint.

Melon and raspberry cups

Serves 4
Each serving: 50 Cals/200 kJ, 10 g (1 unit) carbohydrate, 5 g fibre,
2 g protein, 0 g fat

1 tsp finely grated lemon rind
2 tsp finely grated orange rind
15 ml/1 tbsp lemon juice
120 ml/8 tbsp orange juice

sugar-free liquid sweetener to taste
400 g/14 oz melon, halved and seeded
200 g/7 oz raspberries
mint sprigs

Mix together lemon and orange rind and the juices, add sweetener to taste and leave for 20 minutes.

Scoop the flesh from the melons with a melon baller or cut into large dice. Mix with the raspberries, pour over the juice and mix with the fruit rinds and juices. Then chill for ½ to 1 hour. Spoon back into the melon shells, or a dish, divide the juices between the shells and garnish with the mint sprigs.

Sparkling fruit salad

Serves 4
Each serving: 50 Cals/220 kJ, 10 g (1 unit) carbohydrate, 3 g fibre,
1 g protein, negligible fat

200 g/7 oz apples, cored, but not peeled
115 g/4 oz orange, peeled and seg-mented

60 g/2 oz grapes, halved and de-seeded
425 ml/14 fl oz low-calorie ginger ale
100 g/3½ oz banana

Dice the apples and put into a bowl with the orange segments, grapes and ginger ale. Just before serving slice the bananas and mix with the other fruits. Serve immediately.

Strawberry tartlets   See page 92

Makes 20
Each tartlet: 80 Cals/360 kJ, 10 g (1 unit) carbohydrate, 1 g fibre,
3 g protein, 3 g fat

Pastry:
200 g/7 oz wholemeal flour
100 g/3½ oz cooked mashed potatoes
70 g/2½ oz polyunsaturated margarine
pinch salt

Filling:
400 g/14 oz small strawberries
200 g/7 oz skimmed-milk cheese (see page 35)
300 ml/½ pt prepared strawberry jelly

Heat the oven to 200°C/400°F/gas 6.

Make the pastry (see Vegetable flan au gratin on page 54) and cut into 20 rounds with a fluted cutter. Press into small patty tins and bake for 10–15 minutes. Leave to cool then divide the cheese between them and arrange the strawberries on top. Spoon 15 ml/1 tbsp of jelly, which should be cold and just beginning to set, over the strawberries on each tartlet.

Bramble and apple fluff

Serves 4
Each serving: 80 Cals/340 kJ, 10 g (1 unit) carbohydrate, 8 g fibre,
6 g protein, 2 g fat

200 g/7 oz cooking apples, chopped   *15 g/3 tsp unflavoured gelatine*
200 g/7 oz blackberries, or other   *125 ml/4 fl oz water*
  berries   *2 egg whites, whisked*
sugar-free liquid sweetener to taste   *20 g/2 tbsp chopped hazelnuts*

Cook apples and blackberries together until soft. Add sweetener
to taste. Dissolve the gelatine in 45 ml/3 tbsp hot water and
stir into the fruit. Chill until just beginning to set then fold in
the egg whites stiffly beaten. Pour into a dish and leave to set.
Sprinkle with the nuts before serving.

Summer pudding

Serves 6
Each serving: 120 Cals/500 kJ, 20 g (2 units) carbohydrate, 13 g
fibre, 6 g protein, 1 g fat

680 g/1½ lb blackcurrants or other   *200 g/7 oz sliced wholemeal bread*
  berry fruits   *125 g/4 oz Cream substitute I or II*
125 ml/4 fl oz water   *(see page 105)*
sugar-free liquid sweetener to taste   *few sprigs mint*

Cook the blackcurrants in water for 5–10 minutes until
tender. Allow to cool and add sweetener to taste.
    Remove the crusts from the bread and line a 600-ml (1-pt)
basin or pie dish with 6 slices (cut some of the bread into
triangles to ensure a good fit). Fill with the fruit, cover with the
remaining slice of bread and pour over any juice. Cover with a
plate or piece of polythene, place a weight on top and leave in a
cool place for several hours. Turn out, put spoonfuls of cream
substitute on top and decorate with a few sprigs of mint.

Nutty plum crumble

Serves 4–6
4 servings
Each serving: 190 Cals/810 kJ, 40 g (4 units) carbohydrate, 8 g
fibre, 5 g protein, 4 g fat
6 servings
Each serving: 130 Cals/540 kJ, 20 g (2 units) carbohydrate, 6 g
fibre, 3 g protein, 3 g fat

30 g/1 oz low-fat margarine   *100 g/3½ oz chestnuts, chopped*
100 g/3½ oz wholemeal flour   *680 g/1½ lb plums, halved and stoned*
2 tsp ground cinnamon   *sugar-free liquid sweetener to taste*

Heat the oven to 180°C/350°F/gas 4.

Rub the margarine into the flour and 1 tsp cinnamon. Stir in the nuts. Place half the plums in a baking dish and sprinkle with ½ tsp cinnamon and add sweetener to taste. Cover with approximately one-third of the crumble mixture. Put the rest of the plums on top, sprinkle with ½ tsp cinnamon, and add sweetener to taste. Cover with the remaining crumble mixture and bake for 45–50 minutes.

Black cherry cheesecake

Serves 6

Each serving: 240 Cals/1,000 kJ, 20 g (2 units) carbohydrate, 2 g fibre, 12 g protein, 11 g fat

Base:
100 g/3½ oz digestive biscuits, crushed
45 g/1½ oz polyunsaturated margarine
Filling:
225 g/8 oz skimmed-milk cheese,
  sieved if necessary
300 ml/10 fl oz low-fat plain yoghurt

100 ml/3½ fl oz orange juice (fresh or
  frozen)
15 g/3 tsp unflavoured gelatine
35 g/1 egg white, whisked
sugar-free liquid sweetener to taste
340 g/¾ lb black cherries
10 g/1 tbsp cornflour
30 ml/2 tbsp water

Melt the margarine and thoroughly mix in the biscuit crumbs, press into the base of a flan dish and leave to cool.

Mix together the cheese, yoghurt and orange juice. Dissolve the gelatine in 60 ml/4 tbsp hot water and blend into the cheese mixture. Fold in the egg white and pour onto the base.

Stew the cherries in a little water until beginning to soften. Drain and reserve juice. Remove stones. Blend cornflour and 30 ml/2 tbsp water, add to cherry juice and heat until thickened. Add sweetener to thickened sauce. Stir in fruit. When cool, spread over cheesecake, cover and chill until set.

Apple charlotte

Serves 4

Each serving: 120 Cals/510 kJ, 20 g (2 units) carbohydrate, 4 g fibre, 3 g protein, 4 g fat

340 g/¾ lb cooking apples, cored
115 g/4 oz wholemeal breadcrumbs
sugar-free liquid sweetener to taste

½ tsp (approx) ground cloves or
  cinnamon
30 g/1 oz low-fat spread

Heat the oven to 190°C/375°F/gas 5.

Slice the apples, cross-cut to avoid long pieces of peel and cook in a little water until tender. Add sweetener. Put alternate layers of apples and breadcrumbs in a non-stick pie dish, sprinkling a little spice on each layer. Finish with a layer of breadcrumbs. Dot the top with low-fat spread and bake for 20–25 minutes until brown and crisp.

Apple oatmeal crumble

Serves 4–6
4 servings
Each serving: 230 Cals/950 kJ, 40 g (4 units) carbohydrate, 7 g
fibre, 5 g protein, 7 g fat
6 servings
Each serving: 150 Cals/640 kJ, 20 g (2 units) carbohydrate, 5 g
fibre, 3 g protein, 5 g fat

570 g/1¼ lb cooking apples, cored
¼–½ tsp ground cloves
sugar-free liquid sweetener to taste
60 ml/4 tbsp hot water

30 g/4 tbsp rolled oats
100 g/3½ oz wholemeal flour
30 g/1 oz polyunsaturated margarine

Heat the oven to 180°C/350°F/gas 4.
    Slice the apples in cross-cut slices to avoid long strips of
peel. Place in a baking dish, sprinkle with the cloves, and add
the sweetener to taste. Mix together the oats and flour and rub
in the margarine. Sprinkle over the fruit and bake for 30–40
minutes.
    Other fruits, such as rhubarb or plums, can be used.

Rhubarb charlotte

Serves 4
Each serving: 130 Cals/550 kJ, 20 g (2 units) carbohydrate, 7 g
fibre, 5 g protein, 4 g fat

*450 g/1 lb young rhubarb**
170 g/6 oz wholemeal breadcrumbs
grated rind 1 orange
½ tsp ground ginger
60 ml/4 tbsp orange juice

¼ tsp ground cinnamon and nutmeg
(optional)
sugar-free liquid sweetener to taste
30 g/1 oz low-fat spread

Heat the oven to 190°C/375°F/gas 5.
    Cut rhubarb in 2.5-cm (1-in) lengths and place a layer in a
non-stick pie dish or casserole. Sprinkle a layer of breadcrumbs
on top. Mix together orange rind, ginger, cinnamon and
nutmeg if used, and sprinkle a little over the breadcrumbs.
Repeat the layers, finishing with a layer of breadcrumbs, but
before the final layer pour over the orange juice mixed with
sweetener. Dot the final layer of breadcrumbs with the low-fat
spread. Cover and bake for 20–30 minutes, then uncover and
continue cooking for 10–15 minutes until the top is crisp and
lightly brown. Serve hot.

---

* Older rhubarb may be used, but stew gently with a little water to part-cook before
assembling the pudding.

Cream substitute I

670 Cals/2,830 kJ, 50 g (5 units) carbohydrate, 0 g fibre, 42 g protein, 37 g fat

410 ml/14½ oz can evaporated milk   *30 ml/2 tbsp hot water*
15 g/1½ tsp powdered gelatine   *sugar-free sweetener to taste*

Put gelatine in cup with water and leave for 5–10 minutes to soften. Pour the milk into double saucepan (or a basin placed in a pan of boiling water) and heat until a skin forms. Stir in the gelatine without removing the skin and stir thoroughly until the gelatine has melted.

Pour the mixture into a bowl and when practically cold whisk until stiff. This can be kept for a few days in the refrigerator.

Cream substitute II

190 Cals/820 kJ, 10 g (1 unit) carbohydrate, 0 g fibre, 24 g protein, 6 g fat

150 ml/5 fl oz carton low-fat plain   *15 ml/3 tsp orange or lemon juice*
yoghurt   *sugar-free sweetener to taste*
120 g/4¼ oz low-fat cottage cheese

Mix the ingredients in a blender until smooth and resembling the texture of lightly whipped cream. This can be kept for a few days in the refrigerator.

SNACKS, SAUCES & SALAD DRESSINGS

SNACKS

Red bean pâté

Serves 4
Each serving: 170 Cals/720 kJ, 20 g (2 units) carbohydrate, 5 g fibre, 9 g protein, 8 g fat

100 g/3½ oz wholemeal breadcrumbs   *1 medium-sized onion, chopped*
a little stock   *100 g/3½ oz cooked kidney beans,*
few drops soy sauce   *mashed*
15 ml/1 tbsp corn oil   *60 g/2 oz Edam cheese, grated*

Soak the breadcrumbs in a little stock, adding a few drops of soy sauce. Heat the oil, lightly fry the onion and combine with the beans and cheese, mixing very well. Squeeze most of the moisture from the breadcrumbs and stir into the bean mixture with herbs and seasoning to taste. Chill and serve.

Hummus

Serves 4–6
4 servings
Each serving: 230 Cals/980 kJ, 30 g (3 units) carbohydrate, 8 g fibre, 10 g protein, 10 g fat
6 servings
Each serving: 150 Cals/650 kJ, 20 g (2 units) carbohydrate, 6 g fibre, 7 g protein, 7 g fat

450 g/1 lb canned chick peas (without added sugar), drained
2 cloves garlic, crushed
½ tsp ground cumin
½ tsp salt (or celery salt)
30 ml/2 tbsp corn oil
60 ml/4 tbsp lemon juice
4 tbsp chopped parsley

paprika pepper
4 medium-sized tomatoes, quartered
½ small cucumber, cut in sticks (with skin on)
2 medium-sized carrots, cut into sticks
2 large stalks celery, cut into sticks
340 g/12 oz wholemeal rolls, halved, or wholemeal bread, toasted

Blend or mash the chick peas until smooth and beat in the garlic, cumin and salt. Add spoonfuls of oil and lemon juice alternately, mixing well after each addition. The mixture should have a smooth, firm consistency. Lastly add the parsley, retaining a little for garnish. Adjust seasoning if necessary. Press into a bowl or mould and garnish with the paprika and remaining parsley. Serve with the vegetables and hot wholemeal rolls (or wholemeal bread).

Smoked mackerel pâté

Serves 4
Each serving: 150 Cals/630 kJ, 10 g (1 unit) carbohydrate, negligible fibre, 15 g protein, 9 g fat

200 g/7 oz smoked mackerel, skinned, boned and flaked
100 g/3½ oz skimmed-milk cheese, sieved if necessary (see page 35)

15 ml/1 tbsp French dressing (see page 118)
15 ml/1 tbsp lemon juice
4 ml/1 tsp anchovy essence
seasoning and pinch of nutmeg

Mash together well the mackerel and cheese then thoroughly mix in the remaining ingredients; or mix all ingredients together in a blender. Adjust seasoning and season more highly if liked. Fill into small pots or a mould.

Canned, drained tuna fish, pilchards or salmon may be used instead of the mackerel; and for special occasions, strips of anchovy fillets may be used to garnish.

Bean spread*

Makes 280 g/10 oz
Each 30 g/1 oz: 20 Cals/70 kJ, negligible (0 units) carbohydrate,
1 g fibre, 1 g protein, negligible fat

100 g/3½ oz cooked butter beans
1 shallot or small onion, chopped
½ medium-sized green pepper, chopped

60 g/2 oz unsweetened pickles
30 ml/2 tbsp Lemon and garlic dressing,
well seasoned (see page 118)

Mix all the ingredients in a blender. Spoon into a large bowl or
4 individual bowls and chill.

Black-eyed bean and vegetable spread*

Makes 435 g/16 oz
Each 30 g/1 oz: 20 Cals/70 kJ, negligible (0 units) carbohydrate,
1 g fibre, 1 g protein, negligible fat

100 g/3½ oz cooked black-eyed beans
60 g/2 oz carrot, grated
60 g/2 oz corn kernels
60 g/2 oz leek or onion, chopped
60 g/2 oz red pepper, chopped

60 g/2 oz watercress
30 ml/2 tbsp French dressing (page 118)
seasoning and 1 tsp horseradish sauce

Mix all the ingredients to a fairly smooth paste in a blender.
Spoon into a large bowl or 4 individual bowls and chill.

Trincomalee rice

Serves 6
Each serving: 320 Cals/1,340 kJ, 60 g (6 units) carbohydrate, 6 g
fibre, 14 g protein, 5 g fat

400 g/14 oz long-grain brown rice
1 large onion, finely chopped
seasoning
1 litre/1¾ pts chicken stock, boiling
100 g/3½ oz chicken liver, fried in oil and diced
60 g/2 oz lean cooked ham, diced

60 g/2 oz fresh mushrooms sliced
100 g/3½ oz frozen peas
2 eggs, beaten
100 g/3½ oz pineapple canned in own juice without added sugar, diced
2 tsp soy sauce

Heat the oven to 180°C/350°F/gas 4.
Cook the rice, onion, salt, pepper and stock in a covered
dish in the oven for 1 hour. Stir in the chicken liver, ham,
mushrooms and peas and return to oven for 15 minutes.
Meanwhile, fry the eggs in a non-stick pan and shred finely.
Add to the rice with the pineapple and soy sauce. Lightly fork
through and serve.

---

* It is often simpler to cook larger quantities of beans than stated in the recipes: the
surplus can be kept in the refrigerator for use later in soups, salads etc. Many different
types of beans may be used. Soak, cook and drain according to directions on page 36.

Turkish pilaff

Serves 4–6
4 servings
Each serving: 450 Cals/1,900 kJ, 100 g (10 units) carbohydrate, 11 g fibre, 13 g protein, 3 g fat
6 servings
Each serving: 300 Cals/1,270 kJ, 70 g (7 units) carbohydrate, 7 g fibre, 9 g protein, 2 g fat

400 g/14 oz long-grain brown rice
1 litre/1¾ pts chicken stock, boiling
bouquet garni *(bay leaf, parsley and a sprig of thyme in a muslin bag)*
seasoning

60 g/2 oz currants or raisins, roughly chopped
90 g/3 oz cooked chick peas
1 medium-sized green pepper, chopped
3 medium-sized tomatoes, chopped

Heat the oven to 180°C/350°F/gas 4.

Cook the rice, stock, *bouquet garni*, seasoning, currants or raisins in a covered dish in the oven for 1 hour. Stir in the chick peas, green pepper and tomatoes, cover and cook for 15 minutes. Remove the *bouquet garni* and lightly fork through – it should be dry and flaky.

Try serving it with one of the yoghurt sauces on page 117.

Muesli

Each 60 g/2 oz (dry, without milk or yoghurt): 190 Cals/800 kJ, 30 g (3 units) carbohydrate, 8 g fibre, 6 g protein, 4 g fat

200 g/7 oz rolled oats
60 g/2 oz millet flakes
60 g/2 oz cracked wheat
60 g/2 oz barley flakes
60 g/2 oz rye flakes
60 g/2 oz natural bran flakes

60 g/2 oz dried apricots, chopped
60 g/2 oz dried mixed raisins, currants, sultanas, chopped
60 g/2 oz hazelnuts, chopped
¼ tsp mixed spice

Mix the dry ingredients together and store in an airtight container. Serve with milk or low-fat plain yoghurt or fruit, which may be sweetened with a sugar-free liquid sweetener if liked.

Taken with fresh fruit and skimmed milk or yoghurt, muesli makes a delicious and wholesome snack at any time of the day.

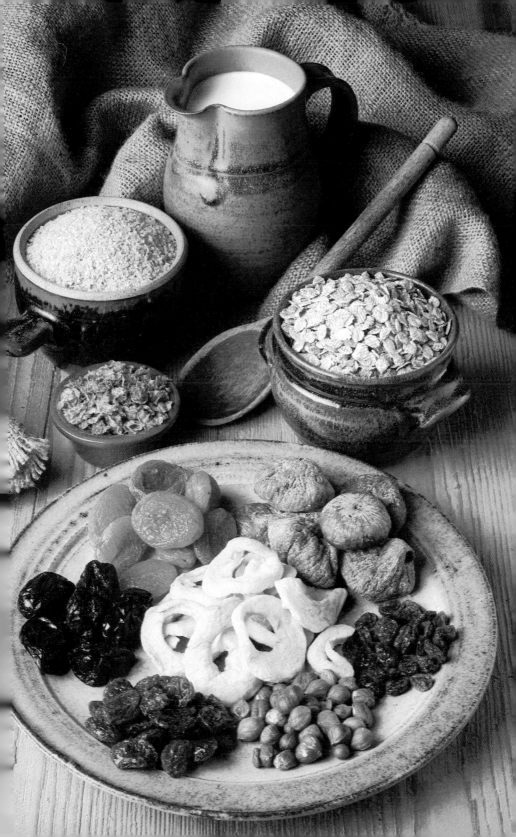

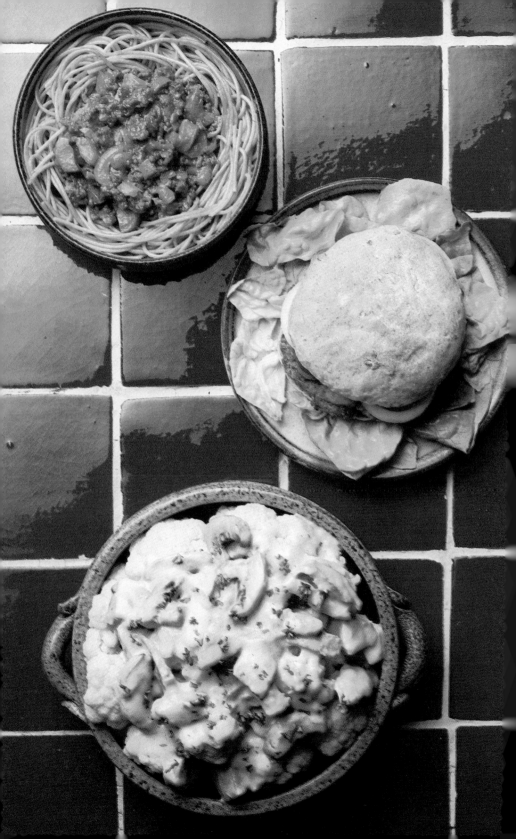

Cauliflower savoury

Serves 4
Each serving: 200 Cals/860 kJ, 10 g (1 unit) carbohydrate, 5 g fibre,
19 g protein, 9 g fat

100 g/3½ oz cooked chicken, cut into small dice
100 g/3½ oz lean cooked ham, chopped finely
225 g/8 oz mushrooms, sliced
1 tsp mild curry powder

500 ml/18 fl oz White sauce (see page 116)
1 large or 2 small cauliflowers, cut into flowerets and including all the leaves and stalk
2 tbsp chopped parsley
seasoning

Add the chicken, ham, mushrooms and curry powder to the sauce and simmer for 10 minutes.

Meanwhile, cook the cauliflower in boiling salted water, drain and put in a flat dish. Pour the hot sauce over and sprinkle with the parsley before serving.

Other seasonings or favourite herbs can be used instead of the curry powder.

Quick paella

Serves 4–6
4 servings
Each serving: 460 Cals/1,920 kJ, 70 g (7 units) carbohydrate, 10 g
fibre, 29 g protein, 8 g fat
6 servings
Each serving: 300 Cals/1,280 kJ, 50 g (5 units) carbohydrate, 7 g
fibre, 19 g protein, 5 g fat

340 g/¾ lb long-grain brown rice
few strands saffron
15 ml/1 tbsp corn oil
1 large Spanish onion, chopped
1 clove garlic, crushed
125 ml/4 fl oz chicken stock
125 g/4 oz fresh or frozen prawns
100 g/3½ oz cooked chicken, diced

115 g/4 oz crab meat
200 g/7 oz peas
1 tbsp sage
seasoning
2 tbsp chopped parsley
1 medium-sized red pepper, cut into strips

Cook the rice (see page 37) with the saffron. Meanwhile, heat the oil and gently fry the onion and garlic until transparent, then add half the stock with the prawns, chicken, crab meat, peas, sage and seasoning. Cook gently until the fish and chicken are hot and the peas are cooked – some of the liquid will evaporate. Stir in the cooked rice adding a little more stock if necessary – the mixture should be slightly moist.
→

Wholemeal spaghetti in meat sauce (*top*, see page 112), Beef and beanburger roll (*centre*, see page 115), Cauliflower savoury (*bottom*).

Lastly, add the parsley and cook for a few minutes.

Low-calorie liver pâté

Serves 4

Each serving: 130 Cals/540 kJ, 10 g (1 unit) carbohydrate, negligible
fibre, 11 g protein, 7 g fat

200 g/7 oz ox liver
1 tbsp celery, chopped
1 tbsp chopped parsley
1 tbsp onion, chopped

150 ml/5¼ oz (½ can) condensed
tomato soup † (alternative flavours
of condensed soup can be used)

Remove veins and skin from the liver and mince finely, then
put the celery, parsley and onion through mincer. Stir into the
soup and cook, beating well, for 10 minutes. Adjust seasoning
and press into a bowl or 4 small pots. Cool, cover and chill.

Wholemeal spaghetti in meat sauce
See page 110

Serves 4

Each serving: 430 Cals/1,810 kJ, 60 g (6 units) carbohydrate, 11 g
fibre, 21 g protein, 12 g fat

30 ml/2 tbsp corn oil
170 g/6 oz lean beef, minced
2 medium-sized onions, chopped
1 clove garlic, crushed
2 medium-sized carrots, chopped
2 sticks celery, chopped

30 ml/2 tbsp tomato purée
375 ml/13 fl oz stock
1 tbsp basil
20 g/2 tbsp chopped peppers
seasoning
340 g/12 oz wholemeal spaghetti

Heat the oil and gently cook the meat, onion, garlic, carrots
and celery for 10 minutes. Stir in the tomato purée, stock,
basil, peppers and seasoning and simmer for 30–40 minutes.

Meanwhile, lower spaghetti gently into a large pan of boiling
salted water and cook for 10–15 minutes or according to
directions on packet. Drain and serve with the sauce on top.

Wholemeal spaghetti with tomato sauce

Serves 4

Each serving: 340 Cals/1,430 kJ, 60 g (6 units) carbohydrate, 10 g
fibre, 13 g protein, 6 g fat

15 ml/1 tbsp oil
1 large onion, chopped
400 g/14 oz canned tomatoes
½ tbsp marjoram

1 tsp garlic salt
pepper
340 g/12 oz wholemeal spaghetti

---

† To make a softer pâté, add 30 ml/2 tbsp extra soup and use as a spread.

Heat the oil and gently fry the onion until pale brown. Stir in the tomatoes and simmer for 15–20 minutes until thickened. Add the marjoram and seasoning.

Meanwhile, boil the spaghetti in salted water for 10–15 minutes or according to directions on packet, then drain well, and serve with the sauce poured over.

Barley and mushroom casserole

Serves 4
Each serving: 470 Cals/1,990 kJ, 80 g (8 units) carbohydrate, 12 g **fibre,** 26 g protein, 9 g fat

15 g/½ oz polyunsaturated margarine
2 medium-sized onions, chopped
1 clove garlic, crushed
450 g/1 lb fresh mushrooms
200 g/7 oz pearl barley
1 tbsp basil
280 ml/½ pt chicken stock
seasoning
200 g/7 oz cold chicken, cut into small pieces
3 tbsp chopped parsley
200 g/7 oz wholemeal spaghetti

Heat the margarine in an oven-proof casserole and gently cook the onion and garlic for 5 minutes until transparent. Stir in the mushrooms and cook slowly for 5 minutes until the mushrooms are golden. Add the barley and basil and toss lightly. Add the stock and seasoning. Slowly bring to the boil, cover, lower the heat and simmer for 30 minutes. Add the chicken, cover and cook for 15–20 minutes until the barley is tender. Meanwhile, cook the spaghetti (see page 38).

Stir the parsley into the casserole and serve with the spaghetti.

Barley pot

Serves 4
Each serving: 500 Cals/2,100 kJ, 90 g (9 units) carbohydrate, 20 g **fibre,** 18 g protein, 12 g fat

15 ml/1 tbsp oil
225 g/8 oz onion, chopped
1 tsp yeast extract
850 ml/1½ pts vegetable stock
60 g/2 oz pearl barley
120 g/4 oz flaked barley
120 g/4 oz haricot beans, soaked (see page 36)
1 bay leaf
1 tbsp marjoram
½ tbsp summer savory
2 cardamom seeds
seasoning
115 g/4 oz fresh or frozen peas
4 medium-sized carrots, grated
30 ml/2 tbsp French dressing (see page 118)
225 g/8 oz wholemeal rolls (see page 93)

Heat the oil and fry the onions until brown. Dissolve the yeast extract in the stock. Add the pearl barley, flaked barley, beans, stock, herbs, cardamom seeds and seasoning to the onion and boil for 10 minutes. Cover and simmer for 2 hours, stirring frequently and adding a little extra stock or water if the mixture becomes too thick. 10 minutes before serving add the peas and adjust seasoning if necessary.

Toss the carrots in the dressing, serve with a side salad, and hand the rolls separately.

Beans in tomato sauce

Serves 4
Each serving: 300 Cals/1,260 kJ, 30 g (3 units) carbohydrate, 9 g **fibre,** 19 g protein, 10 g fat

500 ml/18 fl oz tomato juice	*¼ tsp pepper*
1 shallot or small onion, grated or very	*1 tsp salt*
finely chopped	*pinch dried tarragon*
75 ml/5 tbsp cider vinegar	*450 g/1 lb cooked soya beans (225 g/8*
10 ml/2 tsp Worcester sauce	*oz dry weight)*
dash Tabasco sauce	*200 g/7 oz sliced wholemeal bread,*
¼ tsp celery salt	*toasted (see page 93)*

Boil the tomato juice with the shallot or onion, vinegar, sauces and seasonings for 5 minutes. Remove from the heat, cool, then purée in a blender. Return to the pan, add the beans and cook for 10 minutes. Divide evenly between the slices of toast and serve. (Other medium-sized beans may be used instead.)

Ragout of beans

Serves 4–6
4 servings
Each serving: 280 Cals/1,190 kJ, 40 g (4 units) carbohydrate, 12 g **fibre,** 13 g protein, 9 g fat
6 servings
Each serving: 190 Cals/790 kJ, 30 g (3 units) carbohydrate, 8 g **fibre,** 9 g protein, 6 g fat

30 ml/2 tbsp corn oil	*¼ tsp pepper*
2 large Spanish onions, sliced	*400 g/14 oz cooked butter beans*
2 sticks celery, chopped	*(140 g/5 oz raw weight)*
1 medium-sized carrot, cut in match-	*4 tbsp chopped parsley*
sticks or coarsely grated	*2 tbsp chopped mixed herbs*
25 g/2½ tbsp wholemeal flour	*115 g/4 oz sliced wholemeal bread*
500 ml/1 pt meat or vegetable stock	*toasted, cut in triangles and sprinkled*
1 tsp yeast extract	*with paprika pepper*
1 tsp garlic salt	

Heat the oil and cook the onions, celery and carrots until golden brown, then stir in the flour and brown slightly, stirring. Add the stock, yeast extract and seasonings and stir until boiling. Add the beans and parsley and heat for 10 minutes. Turn onto a large earthenware meat dish, sprinkle the green herbs on top and arrange the toast triangles around the outside.

Hong Kong rissoles

Serves 4
Each serving: 420 Cals/1,750 kJ, 50 g (5 units) carbohydrate, 12 g fibre, 26 g protein, 12 g fat

200 g/7 oz cooked soya beans, minced
200 g/7 oz cooked brown rice
100 g/3½ oz lean cooked ham, minced
1 medium-sized onion, minced
200 g/7 oz corn kernels
2 medium-sized eggs, lightly beaten
75 ml/5 tbsp skimmed milk

200 g/7 oz wholemeal breadcrumbs
3 tbsp chopped parsley
¼ tsp celery salt
¼ tsp pepper
15 ml/1 tbsp lemon juice
paprika pepper
2 bunches watercress or lettuce leaves

Heat the oven to 220°C/425°F/gas 7.

Mix all ingredients together and form into 8 rissoles. Place on a non-stick oven dish and bake for 15–20 minutes until golden brown. Alternatively, cook on each side under a medium-hot grill. Dust with paprika and serve in a border of watercress or lettuce leaves.

Beef and beanburgers

Serves 4
Each serving: 320 Cals/1,340 kJ, 40 g (4 units) carbohydrate, 11 g fibre, 21 g protein, 10 g fat

200 g/7 oz lean minced beef
200 g/7 oz wholemeal breadcrumbs
300 g/10½ oz cooked haricot beans, mashed
1 large onion

2 tbsp chopped parsley
1 tsp garlic salt
¼ tsp pepper
large pinch cayenne pepper
150 ml/5 fl oz skimmed milk

Heat the oven to 190°C/375°F/gas 5.

Mix the meat, breadcrumbs, beans, onion, parsley and seasoning together with a fork. Slowly mix in the milk, divide into 4 and mould into patties. Place on a rack and bake for 20–25 minutes until brown.

Beef and beanburger rolls See page 110

Serves 4
Each serving: 520 Cals/2,200 kJ, 80 g (8 units) carbohydrate, 19 g fibre, 29 g protein, 13 g fat

4 × 85 g/3 oz wholemeal hamburger rolls
4 Beef and beanburgers (see previous recipe)
4 large slices Spanish onion

8 large slices tomato
4 crisp lettuce leaves
4 tbsp Tomato sauce II (see page 117)
4 tbsp dill, gherkin or other sugar-free pickle

Split the rolls, divide ingredients into 4 and fill the rolls.

The salad ingredients may be varied by including sliced cucumber, cress, spring onions or others.

POURING SAUCES

White sauce

Total: 260 Cals/1,080 kJ, 30 g (3 units) carbohydrate, 2 g fibre, 11 g protein, 13 g fat

250 ml/5 fl oz skimmed milk　　*20 g/2 tbsp wholemeal flour*
15 ml/½ oz polyunsaturated margarine　*seasoning*

Put the milk and margarine in a small pan and whisk in the flour. Heat gently, whisking, until the mixture boils and thickens. Cook for 2 minutes then season well.

Variations
Anchovy sauce　Add 10 ml/2 tsp anchovy essence.
Caper sauce　Add 2 tbsp roughly chopped capers.
Parsley sauce　Add 2 tbsp chopped parsley and, if liked, 5 ml/1 tsp lemon juice.

Curry sauce

Total: 510 Cals/2,120 kJ, 50 g (5 units) carbohydrate, 7 g fibre, 7 g protein, 32 g fat

30 g/2 tbsp corn oil　　　　　　　*250 ml/9 fl oz stock*
100 g/3½ oz cooking apple, chopped　*15 g/1 tbsp chutney*
1 medium-sized onion, chopped　　*1 tsp salt*
3 tsp curry powder　　　　　　　*30 ml/2 tbsp lemon juice (or undiluted*
1 tsp curry paste　　　　　　　　*sugar-free squash)*
30 g/3 tbsp wholemeal flour　　　*sugar-free liquid sweetener to taste*

Heat the oil and fry the apple and onion until brown. Add the curry powder and paste and cook gently for 10 minutes. Stir in the flour and cook for a few minutes. Gradually stir in the stock and bring up to the boil. Add the chutney and salt and simmer for 20 minutes. Add the lemon juice and a little sweetener before serving.

Apple sauce

Total: 110 Cals/470 kJ, 30 g (3 units) carbohydrate, 7 g fibre, 1 g protein, 0 g fat

300 g/10½ oz cooking apples, peeled,　*30 ml/2 tbsp water*
*　cored and quartered*　　　　　　*sugar-free liquid sweetener to taste*

Simmer the apples with just enough water to prevent them sticking, until reduced to a pulp, stirring frequently. Sweeten to taste when cool.

Tomato sauce I

Total: 370 Cals/1,550 kJ, 20 g (2 units) carbohydrate, 3 g fibre, 6 g protein, 30 g fat

30 ml/2 tbsp corn oil
1 large Spanish onion, chopped
60 g/2 oz tomato purée
375 ml/13 fl oz water

¼ tsp garlic salt
pepper
pinch mixed herbs

Heat the oil and fry the onion until soft but not brown. Stir in the tomato purée, water, seasonings and herbs. Bring to the boil, stirring, then simmer for 10 minutes, stirring occasionally.

ACCOMPANIMENT SAUCES

These should be used in small amounts so you do not have to include them in your daily calculations.

Tomato sauce II

100 ml/3½ oz low-calorie tomato ketchup
1 tbsp chopped parsley

5 g/1 tbsp chopped capers
1 clove garlic, crushed

Mix all the ingredients together and leave to stand for one hour before serving.

Yoghurt with mandarin dressing

300 ml/10 fl oz low-fat plain yoghurt
20 g/2 tbsp mandarins (canned without added sugar), chopped
30 ml/2 tbsp mandarin juice

½ tsp ground coriander seeds
½ tsp cumin powder
seasoning

Mix all the ingredients together and leave for one hour before serving.

Yoghurt with garlic

300 ml/10 fl oz low-fat plain yoghurt
2 tbsp chopped parsley

seasoning
1 clove garlic, crushed

Mix all the ingredients together and leave to stand for one hour before serving.

DRESSINGS

These should be used in small amounts so you do not have to include them in your daily calculations.

French dressing

60 ml/4 tbsp wine or tarragon vinegar   *½ tsp prepared mustard*
  or lemon juice or a mixture of these   *60 ml/4 tbsp corn or sunflower oil*
½ tsp salt or garlic or celery salt   *2 tbsp chopped herbs (optional)*
¼ tsp pepper

Put all ingredients into a screw-top jar and shake well. Store in the refrigerator.

Tomato dressing

75 ml/3 fl oz sugar-free tomato juice   *¼ tsp celery salt*
30 ml/2 tbsp French dressing (see   *2 tsp Worcester sauce*
  above)   *Large pinch pepper*
¼ tsp garlic salt

Shake all the ingredients together in a screw-top jar. Store in the refrigerator.

Lemon and chive dressing

150 ml/4 fl oz low-fat plain yoghurt   *½ tsp prepared mustard*
1 tbsp chopped chives   *seasoning*
5 ml/1 tsp lemon juice (or sugar-free
  squash)

Mix all ingredients together and chill for ½–1 hour before using.

Lemon and garlic dressing
Omit chives and add ¼ tsp garlic salt.

Yoghurt and tomato dressing

150 ml/5 fl oz low-fat plain yoghurt   *15 ml/1 tbsp sugar-free orange squash*
75 ml/5 tbsp sugar-free tomato juice   *seasoning*
½ tsp Worcester sauce

Mix all ingredients together and chill for ½–1 hour before serving.

APPENDIXES

Appendix 1:
Recommended food list

This appendix is printed in three type styles: normal, **bold** and *italic*. Foods in **bold** type are high in fibre; select as many of these as possible. Foods in *italic* are relatively high in fat; have as few of these as possible. This appendix does not contain foods high in sugar which in our opinion should be taken only on exceptional occasions: when you are ill for example. On occasions when these are needed, their calorie and kiljoule values may be found in appendix 3.

For foods containing appreciable amounts of carbohydrate (CHO), an asterisk* in the appropriate column indicates that the given quantity contains approximately 10 g carbohydrate (1 carbohydrate unit).

All spoon measurements in the appendix are level.

FOOD	WEIGHT	* = 1 CHO unit	Cals/kJ
BREAD			
Wholemeal bread:			
1 thin slice from a small loaf	25 g/¾ oz	*	55/230
½ medium slice from a large loaf	25 g/¾ oz	*	55/230
½ roll	25 g/¾ oz	*	55/230
Chapatis (without fat)	25 g/¾ oz	*	50/210
BISCUITS			
Crispbread, all types (2)	15 g/½ oz	*	60/250
Digestive biscuit (1 large)	15 g/½ oz	*	70/295
Oatcake (1 round)	15 g/½ oz	*	60/280
Plain or semi-sweet biscuits, e.g. cream crackers, rich tea (2)	15 g/½ oz	*	70/295
BREAKFAST CEREALS			
All-Bran (4 tbsp)	25 g/¾ oz	*	70/295

FOOD	WEIGHT	* = 1 CHO unit	Cals/kJ
Bran Flakes; Cornflakes or other sugar-free cereals; **Puffed Wheat (4 tbsp)**	15 g/½ oz	*	55/230
Porridge, made with water (4 tbsp)	120 g/4 oz	*	55/230
Shredded Wheat (½)	10 g/⅓ oz	*	40/170
Weetabix (1)	15 g/½ oz	*	50/210
OTHER CEREALS			
Brown rice, or white, boiled; **wholemeal macaroni,** boiled; white noodles, boiled; **wholemeal spaghetti,** boiled (3 tbsp)	40 g/1⅓ oz	*	50/210
Cornflour; custard powder; **brown rice** or white (dry); sago; tapioca (1 tbsp)	10 g/⅓ oz	*	35/145
Spaghetti, canned in tomato sauce (3 tbsp)	75 g/2½ oz	*	50/210
Wholemeal flour; all other types of wheat flour; cornmeal; **oatmeal; rolled oats; semolina;** (1 tbsp)	15 g/½ oz	*	55/230
Wholemeal or white shortcrust pastry (1 small square)	20 g/⅔ oz	*	115/485
Yorkshire pudding; dumpling (1 small)	40 g/1⅓ oz	*	85/350
VEGETABLES *(see appendix 2 for those which may be eaten freely)*			
Baked beans, canned (4 tbsp)	100 g/3⅓ oz	*	65/275

FOOD	WEIGHT	* = 1 CHO unit Cals/kJ
Beetroot (4 medium slices)	100 g/3⅓ oz *	45/190
Dried beans, boiled, e.g. haricot, red kidney, Mexican, butter or soya beans (2 tbsp)	50 g/1⅔ oz *	50/210
Parsnips, boiled (1 medium)	75 g/2½ oz *	45/190
Peas, canned, processed (3 tbsp)	75 g/2½ oz *	60/250
Peas, dried, boiled (3 tbsp)	50 g/1⅔ oz *	50/210
Potato, boiled or jacket (1 small)	50 g/1⅔ oz *	45/190
Potato, roast (1 small)	50 g/1⅔ oz *	60/250
Sweetcorn, cooked lentils (2 tbsp)	50 g/1⅔ oz *	55/230
FRUIT *(see appendix 2 for those which may be eaten freely)*		
Apple; orange (or 2 tangerines); pear; peach (1 medium)	120 g/4 oz *	50/210
Banana, skinless (1 small)	50 g/1⅔ oz *	40/170
Cherries, fresh, with stones	100 g/3⅓ oz*	40/170
Dates, with stones (2); figs, dried (1 large)	20 g/⅔ oz *	40/170
Fruit juice, unsweetened (1 small glass)	120 ml/4 fl oz*	40/170
Grapes (10)	75 g/2½ oz *	50/210
Plums; apricots, fresh (3 large)	120 g/4 oz *	40/170
Prunes, stewed with stones (4)	50 g/1⅔ oz *	40/170
Strawberries; raspberries	175 g/5⅔ oz *	40/170
Sultanas; raisins; currants (1 tbsp)	15 g/½ oz *	40/170
MEAT		
Corned beef	60 g/2 oz	125/525

FOOD	WEIGHT	* = 1 CHO unit Cals/kJ
Lean bacon, grilled	60 g/2 oz	175/735
Lean beef; lamb; pork, all roast	60 g/2 oz	150/630
Lean chicken; turkey, both roast without skin	60 g/2 oz	140/590
Lean ham	60 g/2 oz	70/295
Kidney; heart; liver, all stewed	60 g/2 oz	100/420
Luncheon meat	60 g/2 oz	185/775
Meat paste	30 g/1 oz	50/210
Sausages, grilled	40 g/1⅓ oz *	125/525
Tongue, boiled	60 g/2 oz	125/525
FISH		
Cockles	60 g/2 oz	30/125
Crab; lobster, both boiled	60 g/2 oz	75/315
Fish fingers; fish cakes, both grilled	60 g/2 oz *	100/420
Fish paste	30 g/1 oz	50/210
Kipper, baked	60 g/2 oz	120/505
Mackerel or herring, grilled	60 g/2 oz	115/485
Mussels	60 g/2 oz	50/210
Pilchards, canned in tomato	60 g/2 oz	75/315
Salmon, canned	60 g/2 oz	95/400
Sardines, canned in oil, drained	60 g/2 oz	125/525
Sardines, canned in tomato	60 g/2 oz	105/440
Shrimps; prawns	60 g/2 oz	60/250
Trout, steamed	60 g/2 oz	80/335
Tuna, canned in oil	60 g/2 oz	175/735
White fish, e.g. cod, haddock, plaice, sole, whiting, baked	60 g/2 oz	55/230
CHEESE		
Cheddar; Cheshire; Emmental; Gruyère	30 g/1 oz	120/505
Cheese spread	30 g/1 oz	90/380
Cottage cheese	30 g/1 oz	30/125
Danish blue	30 g/1 oz	105/440
Edam; Camembert	30 g/1 oz	90/380
Processed cheese	30 g/1 oz	95/400

FOOD	WEIGHT	* = 1 CHO unit Cals/kJ
MILK		
Dried skimmed, without added vegetable fat	20 g/⅔ oz	* 70/295
Evaporated (4 tbsp)	80 ml/3 fl oz	*125/525
Ice cream (1 small brick)	50 g/1⅔ oz	* 80/335
Plain low-fat yoghurt (1 small carton)	150 g/5 oz	* 80/335
Skimmed: fresh; sterilized; longlife	200 ml/⅓ pt	* 65/275
Whole: fresh; sterilized; longlife	200 ml/⅓ pt	*130/545
EGGS		
Boiled or poached (1 medium)	60 g/2 oz	90/380
NUTS		
Almonds	60 g/2 oz	335/1,405
Brazil	60 g/2 oz	370/1,555
Chestnuts	30 g/1 oz	* 50/210
Coconut, fresh	60 g/2 oz	210/880
Hazelnuts	60 g/2 oz	230/995
Peanuts, fresh or roasted	60 g/2 oz	340/1,430
Walnuts	60 g/2 oz	310/1,300
FATS		
Butter	15 g/½ oz	110/460
Low-fat spread	15 g/½ oz	50/210
Margarine	15 g/½ oz	110/460
Vegetable oil	15 g/½ oz	135/570
ALCOHOLIC DRINKS (*see advice on page 34*)		
Beer	250 ml/½ pt	* 90/380
Sherry, dry	75 ml/2½ fl oz	90/380
Spirits (70% proof)	30 ml/1 fl oz	65/275
Vermouth, dry	60 ml/2 fl oz	70/295
Wine, dry	120 ml/4 fl oz	80/335
MISCELLANEOUS		
Bottled brown sauce (4 tsp)	20 g/⅔ fl oz	20/85
Gelatine	30 g/1 oz	95/405

FOOD	WEIGHT	* = 1 CHO unit Cals/kJ
Ovaltine; Bournvita; Horlicks (3 tsp powder)	15 g/½ oz	* 60/250
Thick soup	200 ml/⅓ pt	* 100/420
Tomato ketchup (4 tsp)	20 g/⅔ oz	20/85
Salad cream (2 tbsp)	30 g/1 oz	95/400

Appendix 2:
Free food list

These foods are very low in calories and are therefore allowed freely in all diabetic diets

Vegetables
Asparagus, aubergines, French or runner beans, beansprouts, bamboo shoots, broccoli, Brussels sprouts, courgettes, cabbage, carrots, cauliflower, celeriac, chicory, celery, chives, Chinese cabbage, cucumber, kale, leeks, lettuce, marrow, mushrooms, mustard and cress, onions, parsley, frozen peas, peppers, pumpkin, radishes, spinach, spring greens, tomatoes, turnip, watercress.

Fruit
Blackberries, blackcurrants, lemon, loganberries, gooseberries, grapefruit, rhubarb, redcurrants, melon.

Drinks
Bovril, black tea/coffee, clear soup without thickening or noodles, Marmite, Oxo, sugar-free squashes and Slimline drinks, tomato juice.

Condiments
Clear pickles, curry powder, herbs and spices, mustard, pepper, vinegar, Worcester sauce.

Appendix 3:
'Forbidden' food list

The foods in this appendix are those we would *not* recommend for regular use by diabetics. They are listed for two reasons. First, so that you can count the number of calories you have before changing to our high-fibre diet; and second so that you can count the number of calories you have on exceptional occasions, such as when you are ill or when you take unusual amounts of exercise.

This appendix is not exhaustive. If you need to know the energy values of foods not listed, we would advise you to refer to any reputable calorie-counter booklet, which can be bought at most magazine- or bookstores, or found in public libraries.

	Per 30 g/1 oz Cals/kJ
Apple crumble	60/250
Apple pie with pastry top	50/210
Apple pie, pastry top and bottom	105/440
Bacon (fried): back lean and fat	130/545
streaky lean and fat	140/590
Beefburger, fried	100/420
	Per biscuit
Biscuits: Bourbon cream	70/295
chocolate (fully coated)	125/525
chocolate digestive	130/545
custard creams	70/295
fig roll	60/250
fruit shortcake	35/145
Garibaldi	35/145
Lincoln	45/190
malted milk	40/170
Nice	45/190
Royal Scot	55/230
shortcake	65/275
wafer	45/190
	Per 30 g/1 oz
Black pudding (fried)	85/355
Bread: currant	70/295
malt	70/295
sauce	30/125
soda	75/315
white	65/275
white, fried	160/670

	Per 30 g/1 oz Cals/kJ
Cakes: cheesecake	120/505
currant buns	85/355
doughnuts	100/420
eclairs	105/440
fancy iced cakes	115/485
fruit cake	100/420
gingerbread	105/440
jam tarts	110/460
madeira	110/460
mince pies	125/525
rock cakes	110/460
Victoria sandwich	85/355
Cheese: cream	130/545
Stilton	140/590
Chocolate: fancy and filled	130/545
milk or plain	150/630
	Per bar
Crunchie (large)	165/695
Mars Bar	270/1,135
Milky Way	130/545
Yorkie (milk)	130/545
	Per 30 g/1 oz
Chutney	55/230
Cream: single	65/270
double	135/565
Custard: egg, made with sugar	35/145
made with powder and sugar	35/145
Eggs: fried	70/295
omelette	60/250
Scotch egg	85/355
scrambled	75/315
Faggots	80/335
French dressing (30 ml/1 fl oz)	200/840
Glacé cherries	60/250
Glucose	110/460
Golden syrup	85/355
Haggis (boiled)	95/390
Honey	80/335
Icing sugar	110/460
Jam	75/315
Jelly: packet cubes	75/315
made with water	15/65
made with milk	25/105
Lard	265/1,115
Lemonade (30 ml/1 fl oz)	5/20
Lemon curd	80/335
Liver sausage	95/390

	Per 30 g/1 oz Cals/kJ
Lucozade (30 ml/1 fl oz)	20/85
Marmalade	75/315
Marzipan	125/525
Mayonnaise	215/905
Mincemeat	65/275
Pancakes	90/380
Pastie (Cornish)	95/400
Pastry: flaky, cooked	160/670
shortcrust, cooked	150/630
Pickle, sweet	40/170
Pork pie (individual)	115/480
Potato, chipped	75/315
Potato crisps	160/680
Puddings: bread and butter	45/190
canned rice	25/105
Christmas pudding	85/355
custard tart	80/335
lemon meringue pie	90/380
meringues (no cream)	105/440
milk pudding	35/145
queen of puddings	60/250
sponge pudding	95/400
suet pudding	95/400
treacle tart	105/440
trifle	45/190
Salami	145/620
Sausages (fried)	95/400
Sausage rolls	140/590
Scones	105/440
Steak and kidney pie (individual)	90/380
Suet (shredded)	245/1,035
Sugar: demerara	110/460
white	110/460
Sweets: boiled	95/400
fruit gums	50/210
liquorice allsorts	90/380
pastilles	70/295
peppermints	110/460
toffees	120/505
Treacle (black)	75/315
Yoghurt (fruit flavoured)	25/105

INDEX TO RECIPES

Page numbers in *italics* refer to the illustrations.